T0075003

DIGITAL FUTURE OF HEALTHCARE

DIGITAL FUTURE OF HEALTHCARE

Edited by
Nilanjan Dey, Nabanita Das, and
Jyotismita Chaki

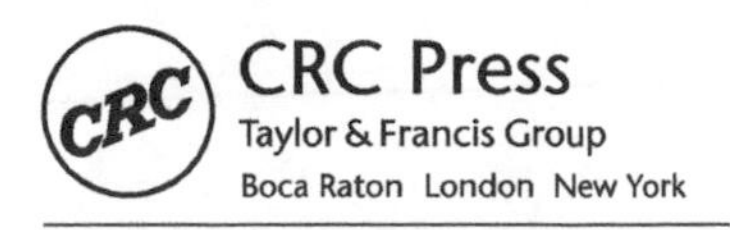

CRC Press is an imprint of the
Taylor & Francis Group, an **informa** business

First edition published 2022
by CRC Press
6000 Broken Sound Parkway NW, Suite 300, Boca Raton, FL 33487-2742

and by CRC Press
2 Park Square, Milton Park, Abingdon, Oxon, OX14 4RN

CRC Press is an imprint of Taylor & Francis Group, LLC

Library of Congress Cataloging-in-Publication Data
A catalog record has been requested for this book

ISBN: 978-1-032-05701-9 (hbk)
ISBN: 978-1-032-05704-0 (pbk)
ISBN: 978-1-003-19879-6 (ebk)

DOI: 10.1201/9781003198796

Typeset in Times
by MPS Limited, Dehradun

Contents

Preface

Digitalization in healthcare services has made an enormous transformation within the healthcare sector over the past few years. The impact of digitalization on the result, quality, and delivery efficiency of healthcare services is obvious by a plethora of examples. Medical professionals have begun to use robotics to perform microsurgery. Besides being a valuable medical education tool, it has resulted in advances in telesurgery and long-distance patient diagnosis (e.g., electrocardiography and computed tomography (CT) scans are often physically performed in one place while the diagnostics are exhausted another). Data analytics, within the medical supply context, can make preparation of pharmaceutical and equipment logistics in hospitals more efficient, while bioprinting (3D printing of organs) and flying drones can help with urgent medical supply needs. Wearable medical devices can facilitate health behavior change, while Internet-based technologies allow fast dissemination of health information. After digitization of the system, it is capable to watch, learn, find out the reason, and act during a practical manner of the acquired data from various perception modalities, like microphones, other sensors. In digitalization systems, machine learning methods and medical analytics are vital tools for extracting significant information. This book presents a comprehensive information of up-to-date requirements in hardware, communication, and calculation for next-generation digitalized healthcare systems. It compares new technological and technical trends and discusses how they address expected digitalized healthcare requirements. A detailed information on various worldwide recent system operations is presented. In particular, challenges in digitalization in healthcare were highlighted. The purpose of this book is not only to help beginners with a holistic approach toward understanding digitalization in healthcare systems but also present to researchers new technological trends and design challenges they have to cope with, while designing such systems. It provides a well-standing forum to discuss the characteristics of digitalization in healthcare in different domains. This book is proposed for professionals, scientists, and engineers who are involved in the technologies typically associated with digitalization in healthcare. This book has several features, including (i) enhancement of the quality of healthcare and make it affordable, (ii) advancement of the healthcare field through exploring digital technologies revolutionize healthcare at the individual, organizational, industry, and societal levels, (iii) it highlights the different techniques, i.e., machine learning, including Internet of Things, medical analytics, and (iv) it includes multi-disciplinary in different applications and challenges with extensive studies on the design, implementation, development, and management of intelligent systems, neural networks, artificial intelligence and related machine learning techniques for digitalization. This book is interesting to specialized analysers to wearable technologies, medical analytics, and statistics. This interdisciplinary domain is related to several domains throughout science and engineering, i.e., computational study, optimization methods, self-organizing feature maps, augmented reality, virtual reality, molecular docking, medical analytics, and statistics.

This book is organized as follows:

Chapter 1 delivers the introduction and some misconceptions about digital healthcare. Also, the state of digital change of healthcare in 2021 and some advantages and challenges of using digital technology in the healthcare industry are discussed in this chapter.

Chapter 2 deals with a novel vision machine technique that has been proposed to diagnose the malignant/highly cancerous and benign/noncancerous skin lesions which are difficult for the radiologists to identify manually in their early stages. This chapter focuses on detecting skin cancer based on various features such as the power spectrum coefficient of DFT, LBP values, variance, and additive fusion of LBP and variance. The detection highly cancerous and noncancerous skin lesions are made using machine learning algorithm like SOM, in which the system is trained based on the history of the skin images stored in the database, and finds the closest match to the current skin image to determine, whether the image under scrutiny is categorized to be highly cancerous or non-cancerous at the initial stage itself. A comparison is made with the various types of distance measures to find the optimal match (minimum distance) using SOM which is a machine learning algorithm.

Chapter 3 is devoted to the recent biomedical applications of wearable devices and sensors in measuring various vital heath parameters and disease diagnosis are discussed along with examples of well-known commercially available wearable devices. Two innovative prototypes which have been developed in house called as RespiroGear – Respiratory Rate Controller and CardioMate-Heart rate and activity monitoring for disease diagnosis have also been described in the present work for the first time.

Chapter 4 is devoted to have an overview of those modern healthcare systems that essentially incorporate the advanced technologies such as IoT, AI&ML, blockchains with their advantages and working limitations. Based on the survey, a cloud-based model is proposed for medical use from an engineering perspective. The abstraction of the model comprises three logical layers for sensing, communicating and processing the data under the centralized control of the M-cloud providing economically and computationally affordable utility to the end users. The model can further be improved by customizing the very needs of the target applications and security concerns.

The chapter considers one of the case studies of novel coronavirus (COVID-19) traces based on its statistical features and detection errors in terms of false positive or false negative margins.

The focus in Chapter 5 is on how to detect epilepsy attack by wireless sensor connected to patient's different body parts. Epileptic patients undergo an unexpected surge of electrical movement in the brain causing a transitory interruption in the messaging systems between the brain cells. The wireless body area sensor locates the body part with seizure movement and will send the signal to the receiver. The comparative study of different algorithm is included in this chapter which shows that Wireless Body Area Sensor is enough efficient for the prediction of epilepsy attack.

Chapter 6 introduce the reader to a case study of surgical assessment and performance prediction within three-dimensional settings by which the healthcare teaching style could be revolutionized. This chapter focuses on clipping Augmented Reality and Machine Learning technologies. A pilot study was conducted, including 14 participants to perform targeting-tasks in three-dimensional space. The participants' performance was measured in a locally developed neurosurgical simulator and based on Fitts' Law. The results indicated that Decision Trees provided less error value in predicting participants' performance than other classifiers.

Chapter 7 deals with an ensemble approach toward argument mining to extract supporting and attacking relationships between sentences from drug reviews, to build an application that can provide a deeper insight into people's opinions on various drugs. The system identifies argumentative content with the presence of discourse indicators, which then undergoes pre-processing and feature extraction. The feature vectors which are extracted from the drug reviews are given to a machine learning classifier for predicting support/attack relations between sentence pairs. A combination of feature sets is considered which consist of structural features, TF-IDF scores for unigrams and bigrams. Three base classification algorithms are evaluated, namely support vector machine, random forest classifier and AdaBoost classifier using precision, recall, F1 scores, and 10-fold cross validation accuracy as evaluation parameters. Further, ensemble methods of voting and stacking are used to improve performance of the existing models.

Chapter 8 presents and analyzes the main researches about augmented reality systems and haptic devices for training of needle insertion, including procedures and target body regions, main devices and physician's evaluation. Using these technologies is a trend in medical training, since it can reduce the training costs and risks involved in procedures, once the medical students can repeat these procedures to exhaustion in a simulated environment before being practiced in a real environment with real people.

The focus in Chapter 9 is on molecular docking study by using AutoDock computational tool, to evaluate the interactions of the phytochemicals like cyclohexane, 1,2,4-triethenyl-, apigenin, and eugenol from tulsi leaves with human cytochromes P450 3A4. Cytochrome P450 3A4 protein is expressed in different organs according to age, and also affects the metabolic function of other proteins. The binding energies of phytochemical with protein were predicted by using molecular docking study and found that the binding energy were -7.9, -10.5, and -7.3 kcal/mol for cyclohexane, 1,2,4-triethenyl-, apigenin, and eugenol, respectively. Based on the observation, the phytochemicals extracted from tulsi leaves can be used in traditional medication to treat various autoimmune and aging disorders.

Chapter 10 deals with the recent progress of the digital health system toward the H2N2 influenza. Much attention was paid to researchers around the world's multi-dimensional approach to design, both hardware and wearable device software, including the application of telemedicine. Digital health systems have therefore been involved in improving different computational technologies in order to overcome the challenges.

Chapter 11 provides an overview of experimentally tested and validated clinical grade CTI images data which were collected from the benchmark dataset and the proposed tool with the KNN classifier helped to attain the better COVID-19 lesion detection

Nilanjan Dey
JIS University
Kolkata, India

Nabanita Das
Bengal Institute of Technology
West Bengal, India

Jyotismita Chaki
Vellore Institute of Technology
Vellore, India

Editors

Nilanjan Dey, PhD. is an Associate Professor in the Department of Computer Science and Engineering, JIS University, Kolkata, India. He is a visiting fellow of the University of Reading, UK. He is an Adjunct Professor of Ton Duc Thang University, Ho Chi Minh City, Vietnam. Previously, he held an honorary position of Visiting Scientist at Global Biomedical Technologies Inc., CA, USA (2012–2015). He was awarded his PhD from Jadavpur University in 2015. He has authored/edited more than 90 books with Elsevier, Wiley, CRC Press, and Springer, and published more than 300 papers. He is the Editor-in-Chief of the *International Journal of Ambient Computing and Intelligence* (IGI Global), Associated Editor of *IEEE Access*, and *International Journal of Information Technology* (Springer). He is the Series Co-Editor of Springer Tracts in Nature-Inspired Computing (Springer), Series Co-Editor of Advances in Ubiquitous Sensing Applications for Healthcare (Elsevier), Series Editor of Computational Intelligence in Engineering Problem Solving and Intelligent Signal Processing and Data Analysis (CRC). His main research interests include medical imaging, machine learning, computer-aided diagnosis, data mining, etc. He is the Indian Ambassador of the International Federation for Information Processing—Young ICT Group and Senior member of IEEE.

Nabanita Das is an Asst. Professor in the Department of Computer Science and Engineering, Bengal Institute of Technology, India. She is currently a Ph.D. Research Scholar with the Department of Computer Science and Engineering, Gandhi Institute of Technology, Orissa, India. She received the M. Tech. degree from MAKAUT, West Bengal, India, and has more than 10 years of teaching experience. She is actively involved in research in the domains of the Machine Learning, IoT, Software Engineering, and Computer-Aided Diagnosis.

Jyotismita Chaki, PhD. is an Assistant Professor in the School of Computer Science and Engineering at Vellore Institute of Technology, Vellore, India. She has done her PhD (Engg) from Jadavpur University, Kolkata, India. Her research interests include: Computer Vision and Image Processing, Pattern Recognition, Medical Imaging, Artificial Intelligence, and Machine learning. She has authored many international conferences and journal papers. She is the author of the following books: *A Beginner's Guide to Image Preprocessing Techniques* (CRC Press 2018); *A Beginner's Guide to Image Shape Feature Extraction Techniques* (CRC Press 2019); *Texture Feature Extraction Techniques for Image Recognition* (Springer 2019); *Image Color Feature Extraction Techniques: Fundamentals and Applications* (Springer 2020); and *Artificial Intelligence for Coronavirus Outbreak* (Springer 2020). She has edited *Smart Biosensors in Medical Care* (Elsevier 2020); and *Sensors for Health Monitoring* (Elsevier 2019), Currently she is the Associate Editor of *Array* journal, Elsevier, *IET Image Processing* Journal (IF: 2.373) and *Machine Learning with Applications*, Elsevier and Academic Editor of PLOS ONE Journal (IF: 3.24).

Contributors

S. Arunmozhi
Department of Electronics and Communication Engineering
Manakula Vinayagar Institute of Technology
Puducherry, India

Abhiruchi Bhattacharya
Department of Computer Engineering
VES Institute of Technology
Chembur, Mumbai, India

Padmaja Borwankar
Department of Computer Engineering
VES Institute of Technology
Chembur, Mumbai, India

Su-Qun Cao
Faculty of Electronic Information Engineering
Huaiyin Institute of Technology
Huaian, Jiangsu

Jyotismita Chaki
School of Computer Science and Engineering
Vellore Institute of Technology
Vellore, Tamil Nadu, India

Cléber Gimenez Corrêa
Universidade Tecnológica Federal do Paraná (UTFPR)
Cornélio Procópio, Brazil

Satya Ranjan Dash
Kalinga Institute of Industrial Technology, Deemed to be University
Bhubaneswar, India

V. Deepti
Department of Electronics and Instrumentation Engineering
St. Joseph's College of Engineering
Chennai, Tamil Nadu, India

Pritam Dhalla
KIIT Technology Business Incubator (KIIT-TBI)
Kalinga Institute of Industrial Technology (KIIT-DU), Deemed to be University
Bhubaneswar, India

Hamza Ghandorh
College of Computer Science and Engineering (CCSE)
Taibah University
Medina, Saudi Arabia

Arpan Ghosh
School of Biotechnology
Kalinga Institute of Industrial Technology, Deemed to be University (KIIT DU)
Bhubaneswar, India

Arpan Ghosh
KIIT Technology Business Incubator (KIIT-TBI)
Kalinga Institute of Industrial Technology (KIIT-DU), Deemed to be University
Bhubaneswar, India

Rajeswari Hari
Department of CSE
SRM Institute of Science and Technology
Chennai, Tamil Nadu, India

Aryan Jaiswal
School of Biotechnology
Kalinga Institute of Industrial Technology, Deemed to be University (KIIT DU)
Bhubaneswar, India

Aryan Jaiswal
KIIT Technology Business Incubator (KIIT-TBI)
Kalinga Institute of Industrial Technology (KIIT-DU), Deemed to be University
Bhubaneswar, India

V. Karthikeyan
School of Biotechnology
Kalinga Institute of Industrial Technology, Deemed to be University (KIIT DU)
Chennai, Tamil Nadu, India

Fahmida Khan
Department of Chemistry
National Institute of Technology
Raipur, India

Sujata Khedkar
Department of Computer Engineering
VES Institute of Technology
Chembur, Mumbai, India

Kasturi Kumbhar
Department of Computer Engineering
VES Institute of Technology
Chembur, Mumbai, India

Ariscia Mendes
Department of Computer Engineering
VES Institute of Technology
Chembur, Mumbai, India

Biswajit Mishra
School of Applied Sciences
Kalinga Institute of Technology (KIIT), Deemed to be University
Bhubaneswar, India

Namrata Misra
School of Biotechnology
Kalinga Institute of Industrial Technology, Deemed to be University (KIIT DU)
Bhubaneswar, India

Namrata Misra
KIIT Technology Business Incubator (KIIT-TBI)
Kalinga Institute of Industrial Technology (KIIT-DU), Deemed to be University
Bhubaneswar, India

Nirmal Kumar Mohakud
Department of Pediatrics
Kalinga Institute of Medical Sciences, KIIT Deemed to Be University
Bhubaneswar, India

Maheswata Moharana
School of Applied Sciences
Kalinga Institute of Technology, Deemed to be University
Bhubaneswar, India

Claiton de Oliveira
Universidade Tecnológica Federal do Paraná (UTFPR)
Cornélio Procópio, Brazil

Subrat Kumar Pattanayak
Department of Chemistry
National Institute of Technology
Raipur, India

T. Pavithra
Department of Electronics and Instrumentation Engineering
St. Joseph's College of Engineering
Chennai, Tamil Nadu, India

R.S. Ponmagal
Department of EEE
Dr. MGR Educational & Research Institute
Chennai, Tamil Nadu, India

V. Rajinikanth
Department of Electronics and Instrumentation Engineering
St. Joseph's College of Engineering
Chennai, Tamil Nadu, India

Mayur Rathi
Walchand College of Engineering
Sangli (MS) India

Ratula Ray
Classes and Technologies
Kalinga Institute of Industrial Technology, Deemed to be University
Durgapur, West Bengal, India

Rahul Roy
Classes and Technologies
Durgapur, West Bengal, India

Rojalin Sahu
School of Applied Sciences
Kalinga Institute of Technology (KIIT), Deemed to be University
Bhubaneswar, India

Satya Narayan Sahu
School of Applied Sciences
Kalinga Institute of Technology (KIIT), Deemed to be University
Bhubaneswar, India

Satya Narayan Sahu
Hydro & Electrometallurgy Department
CSIR-Institute of Minerals and Materials Technology
Bhubaneswar, India

Silvio Ricardo Rodrigues Sanches
Universidade Tecnológica Federal do Paraná (UTFPR)
Cornélio Procópio, Brazil

Vaddi Satya Sai Sarojini
Department of Information Technology
St. Joseph's College of Engineering
Chennai, Tamil Nadu, India

Alo Sen
Classes and Technologies
Durgapur, West Bengal, India

S.P. Sonavane
Walchand College of Engineering
Sangli (MS), India

S.P. Sonavane
V. J. T. I Matunga
Mumbai, India

Mrutyunjay Suar
School of Biotechnology
Kalinga Institute of Industrial Technology, Deemed to be University (KIIT DU)
Bhubaneswar, India

Mrutyunjay Suar
KIIT Technology Business Incubator (KIIT-TBI)
Kalinga Institute of Industrial Technology (KIIT-DU), Deemed to be University
Bhubaneswar, India

K. Sujatha
Professor, Dept. of EEE, Dr. MGR Educational & Research Institute
Chennai, Tamil Nadu, India

V. Srividhya
Department of EEE
Meenakshi College of Engineering
Chennai, Tamil Nadu, India

K.S. Thivaya
Department of ECE
Dr. MGR Educational & Research Institute
Chennai, Tamil Nadu, India

Varsha Varghese
Department of Electronics and Instrumentation Engineering
St. Joseph's College of Engineering
Chennai, Tamil Nadu, India

1 Introduction to Digital Future of Healthcare

Jyotismita Chaki
School of Computer Science and Engineering, Vellore Institute of Technology, Vellore, Tamil Nadu, India

CONTENTS

1.1 INTRODUCTION

Digitalization in healthcare has adopted the same trend as other sectors. In the 1950s, as organizations began using modern digital technologies to simplify extremely structured and routine processes such as billing and accounting, healthcare payers began to use information technology to process massive volumes of statistical evidence [1–3]. Two decades later, the second phase of digitization is here. It has done two things: it has helped merge various aspects of the central processes within individual organizations, and it has assisted B2B processes like supply chain management for different agencies within and beyond individual sectors. As far as

DOI: 10.1201/9781003198796-1

its influence on the healthcare industry is concerned, this second phase of digital implementation has helped develop, for example, an electronic health card.

Members in the healthcare sector were moderately benefitted after the first and second waves of digitalization. But they failed to effectively handle the various stakeholders, policies, and privacy issues needed to create a truly integrated digitized healthcare system. This is partly because the first and second waves of digitalization concentrated more on procedures rather than on patient needs.

Now that patients across the world have become more relaxed with digital networks and resources, including for complicated and delicate matters such as healthcare (popular sites like Zocdoc [4], Tia [5], Flutter Health [6] are only three instances of this trend), the time has come for the digitalization of healthcare services.

1.2 MISCONCEPTIONS OF DIGITAL HEALTHCARE

Excellence in the third wave of digitalization relies mostly on first realizing the digital needs of patients in both the network and the facility [7,8]. Yet many digital health practices are also guided by misconceptions or evidence that are no longer relevant. This chapter highlights four of those perspectives.

1.2.1 Misconception 1: People Do Not Want to Adopt Automated Healthcare Services

Many healthcare providers claim that, due to the delicate nature of the medical treatment, people do not choose to use digital services except in a few special cases; decision-makers also invoke statistics that suggest a comparatively poor use of digital health services. Currently, the findings show something different [9]. The reason is patients are reluctant to embrace digital healthcare as current methods do not satisfy their needs or are poor in quality. Patients would like to utilize digital healthcare facilities if those facilities encounter their desires and deliver the excellence level they imagine. Of course, nondigital channels will continue to be relevant and important, so digital channels will have to be embedded in a well-thought-through multichannel concept.

1.2.2 Misconception 2: Mainly Young Adults Choose Digital Services

One of the most common misconceptions around healthcare is that only young adults choose to utilize digital services, and hence digital healthcare does not meet several of the system's main stakeholders. However, the main situation is that patients of all age categories can utilize automated healthcare systems. Elderly patients want automated healthcare facilities just as much as their younger individuals [10]. There is a variation, however, between the types of digital platforms that elderly and young patients are using. Elderly patients favor conventional digital platforms like sites and e-mails, whereas younger patients are predictably more responsive to newer platforms like social networking. The program level, not only the platform, should be partitioned by age; younger patients, of course, prefer to access health promotion and preventive programs, while elderly patients prefer data about urgent and chronic care services. But both parties are finding information at the same time.

1.2.3 Misconception 3: Mobile Health or M-health Is a Game-changer

M-health, the study of treatment enabled by mobile devices, is also celebrated as the direction of digital healthcare services. However, the availability of mobile healthcare is not widespread. It is also not the only important part of the future of healthcare digitalization.

There is a market for M-healthcare apps, and it is the highest among younger patients [11]. Health services should also build mobile applications that address these customers, for instance, infant health applications or those that may be categorized as fitness applications. Digital technologies can treat chronic problems that are usually seen in older adults.

1.2.4 Misconception 4: Patients Are Searching for New Applications and Features

Healthcare systems, payers, and suppliers also feel that they desire to be creative when developing their digital service contributions. But the key features people desire from their healthcare system are shockingly trivial: quality, easier access to information, compatibility with other platforms, and the accessibility to a real person if the digital service does not offer them what they want and need. Extremely developed technology, better applications, and more social networks are much less relevant for most patients.

1.3 THE STATE OF DIGITAL CHANGE OF HEALTHCARE IN 2021

To recognize its meaning, it is important to consider the assumptions and facts of what patients need from digital healthcare. Thanks to innovations, patients are better treated with augmented reality equipment, wearable technologies, telehealth, and 5G digital technology. Doctors, on either hand, will automate their workflows by using Artificial Intelligence.

Here is a closer look at the state of digital change of healthcare in 2021:

1.3.1 The Growth in On-Demand Healthcare (Why Patients Need Healthcare on Their Schedule)

When thinking of "on-demand," one may think of customers who desire things for their comfort, at their period wherever they appear to be. Healthcare is approaching the age of digitalization when patients are opting for on-demand healthcare due to their heavy workload. Mobile is particularly relevant when considering digital marketing.

People have become much more responsive to the digital era in the past decade. Mobility is the key to success, and recent figures indicate that most of the web surfing in the world takes place on smartphones [12].

Among the first principles for digital marketing is that people need to understand where the targeted audiences are coming together and approach them on those channels, that is, smartphones. This is not shocking considering that 77% of Indian citizens own a mobile.

More than four billion people worldwide are on the Internet, and there is a need for digitalization in healthcare.

Potential customers went online to access patient files for the following reasons:

- 47% of research physicians
- 38%research hospitals and healthcare facilities
- 77% book hospital appointments

The online market that connects physicians directly to healthcare facilities for short-term work makes things simpler for doctors to offer on-demand medical care to patients in particular circumstances that fit their skills, knowledge, and availability. In other words, physicians themselves become on-demand healthcare providers to adequately meet the changing requirements of the clients, another advantage of digitalization in the healthcare sector.

1.3.2 The Significance of Big Data in the Health Industry

Big data consolidate business information across platforms like social networking sites, e-commerce, online purchases, and banking transactions, and detect patterns and trends for potential usage [13].

Big data offers a range of significant features for the healthcare industry, which includes the following:

- **The lower level of medical error**: Via medical record review, the software will highlight any discrepancies between a patient's healthcare prescriptions, alerting health practitioners and patients whenever there is a possible risk of a drug error.
- **Promoting preventive treatment**: A significant number of people visiting emergency departments. Big data analysis could classify these individuals and make protective intends to continue them from returning.
- **More reliable staffing**: A large data predictive analysis might allow clinics and hospitals to forecast potential admission rates, which enables these facilities to assign adequate personnel to the care of patients. This saves a lot of money and reduces the waiting time in the emergency department when the hospital is short-staffed.

With these advantages in mind, pharmaceutical and medical companies should participate in the organization of their data. This refers to the investment in analytics specialists who can integrate data not just to find weak points, but to also help organizations better understand their business.

1.3.3 The Wonder and Care of Patients with Artificial Intelligence

Ten years ago, telling people that they could reduce their suffering with a computer game-like gadget would have received a lot of empty stars. Now Artificial Intelligence is a part of the resistance to digitalization in healthcare [14]. Its multitude of applications is rapidly changing the way patients are viewed.

Artificial Intelligence is much more than a pattern of digitalization in healthcare. Artificial Intelligence is the ultimate example of medical advancement, and industry leaders are willing to invest millions in it. Almost all aspects of the industry will be influenced by this application.

Most of the patients relate Artificial Intelligence in medicine to the Japanese nurse robots. And now there are several American variants, like Moxi, a friendly hospital robot programmed to assist human nurses with basic activities like recovery and extraction of medication.

Chatbots and virtual health helpers are yet another Artificial Intelligence-based technologies that patients are comfortable with. Chatbots can perform a wide variety of roles from salespeople to diagnostic tools and even clinicians. Their flexibility is converted into substantial investment.

But the actual power of Artificial Intelligence can best be seen in fields such as new treatments, computer vision, drug development, and cell biology. For example, cancer patients are required to undergo high-failure cookie-cutter therapies. Now, kudos to Artificial Intelligence's advanced pattern recognition, these patients have access to customized therapy based on their genetic structure and behavior.

What Artificial Intelligence-powered computer algorithms do for oncology, in a summary, is to examine thousands of pathological images of different cancers to deliver highly accurate diagnoses and determine the best suitable combinations of anticancer drugs. And, in radiology diagnostics, Artifical Intelligence-based devices allow radiologists to identify information that bypasses the human visual system.

Moreover, top biotechnology and pharmaceutical firms use machine learning techniques to reduce the time of drug development.

1.3.4 Development of Wearable Healthcare Devices

Another pattern of digitalization in healthcare is that businesses gather their medical data from medical equipment, particularly wearable devices [15]. In the past, numerous patients were pleased with physical exercise once per year and only checked in along with their physicians if something went wrong. However, in the digital era, patients are more likely to concentrate on safety and prevention and to seek more information on their health.

As a consequence, healthcare providers are involved in engaging in wearable technology systems that provide up-to-date tracking in high-risk patients to assess the probability of a major health incident.

Some of the most popular devices are:

- Heart rate monitors
- Activity trackers

- Sweat meters are used by diabetics to monitor and control blood sugar levels
- Oximeters measure the amount of oxygen carried in the blood and are frequently used in patients with respiratory disorders like COPD or asthma

1.3.5 Blockchain and the Future of Improved Electronic Medical Records

Blockchain has recently developed a bad reputation due to the collapse of crypto currency market. Now, the average individual considers blockchain an abstract, confusing idea that does not have much impact on individuals [16,17]. This technology will eventually play a critical role in ensuring their electronic medical records consistent and protected.

Blockchain is a distributed ledger or a computerized transaction database. Shared through a computer network, it enables consumers to share banking details securely with manufacturers with no need for a third party, including a bank.

The pharmaceutical and healthcare industries are already committed to their productivity by investing millions in this business.

An electronic medical record is simply the digital version of the medical record which contains everything from health history and diagnosis to treatment, vaccination dates, and test results. It also includes their home address, former workplaces, and also financial data like credit card information.

1.4 ADVANTAGES OF DIGITAL HEALTHCARE

Some advantages of digital health are as follows [18–20]:

1. Digital health makes healthcare available in difficult-to-reach regions. Through an Internet link, everyone can obtain health services and still be linked to a doctor to address issues.
2. The doctor can preserve all the appropriate information, view it when he or she needs it, and share it with the patient or other medical practitioners. The data would assist in making more detailed reports, compare patient progress to ensure treatment judgment more effectively.
3. Interactive innovations contribute to improved clinical practice and commitment to care due to the biofeedback they obtain in real-time. ReHub is an instance of dedication to digitalization in the healthcare system. It is the first digital approach for physical neurological rehabilitation that helps patients exercise whenever and wherever they choose, while the specialist tracks their progression at all times.
4. With longer lifespans, an increasing number of patients suffering from chronic diseases, and rising healthcare costs, there is an ever-increasing burden on healthcare systems worldwide. There is also an increasing move toward digital health strategies. With digital health systems, patients have faster access to healthcare services with high-quality treatment. Concurrently, these networks allow reducing the pressure on healthcare services by promoting the concept of patient self-care.

5. Digital health systems allow patients to self-manage their health problems by tracking and recording their symptoms daily. More specifically, it is a tool for early identification of major changes in the course of the disease in a patient until the health has been irrevocably impaired. Digital health channels are therefore of great importance for patients with chronic illnesses who are at risk.
6. Digital health services connect patients with their physicians, allowing them to become co-designers of their treatment and care strategies. Rapid, straightforward, and reciprocal exposure to the patient's current health condition improves the sense of collaboration, confidence, and openness between the patient and the physician. Significant factors influencing health, like time of day, atmospheric stimulants, the use of medicines, and tolerance to drugs, can all be recorded in real-time and can be utilized to provide a consistent overview of the condition of the patient.
7. Digital health technologies help minimize the logistical burden of health practitioners and other tedious aspects of their work. This improves their time for real patient-contact and supervision. This is especially relevant for patients or hospitals located in remote areas or for residential or out-patient travel that is challenging or not prescribed. With clinical-grade technology, patients are ready to send their health records to their doctors at any time.
8. The availability of accessible medical technology in hospitals decreases the economic burden of disease control for both laboratories and patients. Many virtual care networks are also a gateway to online forums where patients can find support and interaction with others on related diseases.

1.5 CHALLENGES IN DIGITAL HEALTHCARE

Some challenges in digital healthcare are as follows [21,22]:

1. Health practitioners often feel challenged by the use of emerging technologies. However, digitalization should be seen as a tool that complements the quality of service and not as a substitute and also allowing them to maximize their time.
2. Every technical advance contributes to work on research and development. Sometimes this can be expensive, but there is still no desire to compensate, both on the part of public authorities as well as on the part of patients.
3. The collection and interpretation of data is a big problem for the healthcare sector. Part of the issue is the vast volume of data that clinics, health center practitioners are gathering. Without a reliable Artificial Intelligence system that can evaluate this data, it is difficult for organizations to offer quality and more personalized treatment to patients. Collecting and synchronizing data is another big obstacle. As telemedicine increases, physician visits are taking place through various networks, making it more difficult for health practitioners to monitor patient medical records. As a consequence, it will be important for the healthcare system to develop a way to monitor and maintain medical records for both in-person and online appointments.

4. Cybersecurity is a problem for every sector, and the healthcare system is no exception. Companies must remain extremely cautious against cyber attacks, which can be incredibly expensive. For instance, the IBM study found that healthcare companies lost huge revenue due to data attacks, which were three times higher than other sectors. In healthcare, the three most popular weaknesses are user authentication failures, network leakage, and improper user permissions. Appropriate steps to improve these areas are important to the protection of the healthcare sector. Moreover, the introduction of digital devices and the overall digitalization of the industry are likely to lead to more threats. Digital devices can face difficulties when it comes to safety-related components that manufacturers can stop supporting after a certain amount of time. While threats may come from those seeking damage, others may result from errors in the development of a product or software. Software-producing companies, mobile apps, websites, digital devices, etc. must ensure that vulnerabilities like these are found and addressed before products and services are released or upgraded.
5. Last but not least, developing devices such as a connected heart rate monitors, smartphone apps, or any other digital services or products that work perfectly and are user-friendly is a significant challenge. When it relates to any sort of technology, attention must be provided to the end customer to meet customer requirements or product that is pleasant to use. This is particularly relevant in the healthcare field, as many goods can be utilized by both patients and doctors. An inconvenient or poorly built digital system, for instance, can spoil the patient's experience and allow them to uninstall a device that limits the data they can gather. On the other hand, if the software is hard to use, the general desire of health personnel to use or recommend the technology to other patients would also be reduced. The lack of responsibility, specifically when it comes to digital devices, makes it increasingly challenging for these services and products to work perfectly in an environment of devices that are connected. However, the potential of technology to introduce significant changes in the healthcare sector will ultimately depend on its overall performance.

1.6 SUMMARY

This chapter presents an overview of the digital future of healthcare. With technology making rapid progress every day, it is very clear that the future of healthcare will rely primarily on digital automation. Health practitioners will need to learn a variety of new skills that are required, such as how to use this modern technology and how to efficiently provide virtual appointments, diagnostics, and care therapies. Healthcare experts will also need to learn how to interpret the data from patient wearable devices, digital healthcare records, and genome, to identify, assisted by Artificial Intelligence innovations to improve performance. Wearables implanted under the skin will test blood for viruses, toxins, and bacteria. The data obtained by these implants will be communicated with the health-related app, digital health tracking subscription service, or local healthcare network to alert the patient of an imminent infection before the patient experiences any symptoms.

If these developments become more popular, we need to understand what it means during the next century of medical equipment and systems. As developers, we need to push ourselves to guarantee that innovative technologies and services meet real existing challenges and allow organized patient-centered support to improve better outcomes. The digital future of healthcare will have to promote performance and understanding and strengthen the effectiveness and role of medical practitioners rather than substitute human contact and demeaning treatment. Although technology can and will allow improved results, it is important to keep the needs of patients and consumers at the forefront of our thoughts to ensure that healthcare professionals can do much better.

REFERENCES

1. Biesdorf, S., & Niedermann, F. (2014). *Healthcare's digital future*. McKinsey & Company, London.
2. Dal Mas, F., Piccolo, D., Edvinsson, L., Skrap, M., & D'Auria, S. (2020). Strategy innovation, intellectual capital management, and the future of healthcare: The case of Kiron by Nucleode. In *Knowledge, people, and digital transformation* (pp. 119–131). Springer, Cham.
3. van der Zande, M. M., Gorter, R. C., & Wismeijer, D. (2013). Dental practitioners and a digital future: An initial exploration of barriers and incentives to adopting digital technologies. *British Dental Journal*, *215*(11), E21.
4. Zocdoc (https://www.zocdoc.com/)
5. Tia (https://asktia.com/)
6. Future Health (https://www.flutterhealth.com/)
7. Willems, E. (2019). The digital future. In *Cyberdanger* (pp. 185–199). Springer, Cham.
8. Garcia-Ruiz, M. A., Tashiro, J., Kapralos, B., & Martin, M. V. (2011). Crouching tangents, hidden danger: Assessing development of dangerous misconceptions within serious games for healthcare education. In *Virtual immersive and 3D learning spaces: Emerging technologies and trends* (pp. 269–306). IGI Global, Hershey, Pennsylvania.
9. Digital health customer survey (https://www.accenture.com/us-en/insights/health/leaders-make-recent-digital-health-gains-last)
10. Seniors are online now (https://www.weforum.org/agenda/2019/07/no-longer-just-for-the-young-70-of-seniors-are-now-online/)
11. M-Health (https://www.gminsights.com/industry-analysis/mhealth-market#:~:text=mHealth%20Market%20size%20was%20valued,CAGR%20from%202019%20to%202025.&text=Emerging%20technologies%20in%20support%20of,in%20the%20recent%20past%20years)
12. Web Surfing (https://www.broadbandsearch.net/blog/mobile-desktop-internet-usage-statistics)
13. Importance of big data in healthcare (https://www.optisolbusiness.com/insight/importance-of-big-data-in-healthcare)
14. Davenport, T., & Kalakota, R. (2019). The potential for artificial intelligence in healthcare. *Future Healthcare Journal*, *6*(2), 94.
15. Lee, G. H., Moon, H., Kim, H., Lee, G. H., Kwon, W., Yoo, S., Myung, D., Yun, S. H., Bao, Z., & Hahn, S. K. (2020). Multifunctional materials for implantable and wearable photonic healthcare devices. *Nature Reviews Materials*, *5*(2), 149–165.

16. Gordon, W. J., & Catalini, C. (2018). Blockchain technology for healthcare: Facilitating the transition to patient-driven interoperability. *Computational and Structural Biotechnology Journal*, *16*, 224–230.
17. Zhang, P., Schmidt, D. C., White, J., & Lenz, G. (2018). Blockchain technology use cases in healthcare. In *Advances in computers* (Vol. 111, pp. 1–41). Elsevier.
18. Edirippulige, S., & Senanayake, B. (2020). Professional practices for digital healthcare. In *Opportunities and challenges in digital healthcare innovation* (pp. 97–112). IGI Global, Hershey, Pennsylvania.
19. Rantala, K. (2018). Professionals in value co-creation through digital healthcare services. *Jyväskylä Studies in Business and Economics*, (189) ISBN: 978-951-39-7454-1.
20. Ma, Y., Zhang, Y., Cai, S., Han, Z., Liu, X., Wang, F., Cao, Y., Wang, Z., Li, H., Chen, Y., & Feng, X. (2020). Flexible hybrid electronics for digital healthcare. *Advanced Materials*, *32*(15), 1902062.
21. Brown, I., & Adams, A. A. (2007). The ethical challenges of ubiquitous healthcare. *The International Review of Information Ethics*, *8*, 53–60.
22. Medhekar, A., & Nguyen, J. (2020). My digital healthcare record: Innovation, challenge, and patient empowerment. In *Opportunities and challenges in digital healthcare innovation* (pp. 131–150). IGI Global, Hershey, Pennsylvania.

2 A Content-Based Image Retrieval System for Diagnosis and Detection of Skin Cancer Using Self-Organizing Feature Maps

K. Sujatha[1], R.S. Ponmagal[1], Rajeswari Hari[2], M. Anand[1], V. Karthikeyan[3], V. Srividhya[4], N.P.G. Bhavani[5], and Su-Qun Cao[6]

[1]Department of EEE, Dr. MGR Educational & Research Institute, Chennai, Tamil Nadu, India
[2]Department of CSE, SRM Institute of Science and Technology, Chennai, Tamil Nadu, India
[3]Department of Biotechnology, Dr. MGR Educational & Research Institute, Chennai, Tamil Nadu, India
[4]Department of ECE, Dr. MGR Educational & Research Institute, Chennai, Tamil Nadu, India.
[5]Department of EEE, Meenakshi College of Engineering, Chennai, Tamil Nadu, India.
[6]Faculty of Electronic Information Engineering, Huaiyin Institute of Technology, Huaian, Jiangsu China

CONTENTS

DOI: 10.1201/9781003198796-2

2.1 INTRODUCTION

The skin is the largest exposed organ which covers the entire body. It serves as a part of the excretory system that helps eliminate sweat from the body. This exposed region of the skin is called the epidermis and the layer underneath this is called the dermis. The skin is made of three different varieties of cells, namely, the squamous cells, basal cells, and melanocytes. Skin cancers are developed due to exposure to Ultra-Violet (UV) radiation which causes changes in the genetic material, namely the DNA composition. People with more number of moles, dark skin, fair skin, freckled skin, or even heredity are affected by melanoma [1–4]. The cross section of the skin is shown in the Figure 2.1.

Skin cancers begin in the pigment-containing cells called as melanocytes and the pigment is called as melanin. The cancerous cells in basal cell carcinoma and squamous cell carcinoma do not lead to development of melanomas, and hence are called the non-melanoma skin cancers. Usually melanomas are brown, black, blue, red, or even colorless. They grow on any part of the skin which is largely exposed to sun and are most likely to be found on the neck, face, trunk, and legs. The squamous and basal cell carcinomas are dangerous, because these are very difficult to identify from the normal and abnormal squamous and basal cells at their early stages. If detected at their early stage, the spreading of the cancerous cells on the skin can be inhibited by appropriate treatment [5–10]. Basal cell skin cancers can attack bones and other tissues under the skin and once cured can also reoccur on the same portion of the skin. Squamous cell skin cancers attack the tissues below the skin and spread to the lymph nodes. Hence, squamous cell skin cancers are more dangerous than basal cell skin cancers [11–15].

The major causes of skin cancers could be the treatment for psoriasis, xeroderma pigmentosum (XP), basal cell nevus syndrome, smoking, HPV infection, and reduced immunity. Figure 2.2(a), shows a normal mole on the face whereas Figure 2.2(b) depicts the various forms of melanoma present on the skin. Generally, dermatologists adapt the “abcde” rule to classify patches on the skin [16–20].

“a” = Asymmetry indicates irregularity color and structure of skin
“b” = Boundary denotes the characteristics of the boundary
“c” = Color variation specifies the nonuniform nature in the spread of pigments
“d” = Diameter should be more than 6 mm in size
“e” = development or new start of a blister

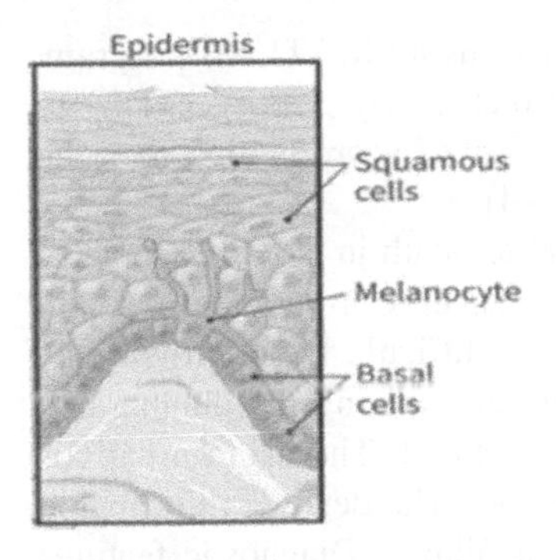

FIGURE 2.1 Cross Section of Skin.

2.2 RESEARCH HIGHLIGHTS

- A highly cancerous growth on various regions of the skin can be diagnosed using vision machine techniques so as to offer an error-free diagnosis.
- Local Binary Pattern (LBP) is used to represent the images of skin and develop a retrieval system that matches and retrieves images with the support of the LBP operator.
- Similarity measurement is done by many methods like L1 or Manhattan distance measure, Euclidean distance measure or L2, d_1 distance measure, and Canberra distance measures. The selection of distance measure affects the similarity metrics and greatly influences the retrieval performance.
- Enhanced clustering for categorization of noncancerous and highly cancerous skin blisters is done using SOM.

2.3 REVIEW ON SKIN CANCER

The most deadly type of skin cancer is the malignant melanoma, which when screened at an early stage can be efficiently treated and cured. Surgical expurgation is an efficient way to remove the melanoma. To increase the efficiency of diagnosis by dermatologists, computer-aided vision methods are used. Some simple image-

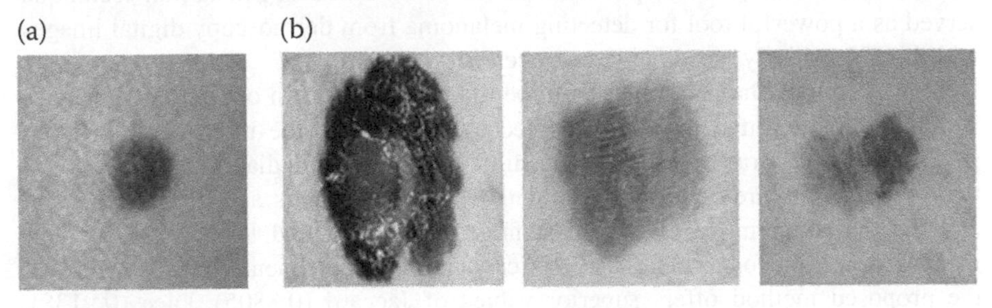

FIGURE 2.2 Images of Patches on the Skin (a) Normal mole on the face, (b) Various forms of melanoma present on the skin. From (http://www.dermquest.com)

processing algorithms are used to detect the skin cancer using MATLAB program, which is used to calculate the "VXYZ" (Total Dermatoscopy Score – TDS) to detect the potentially malignant melanomas. If the "VXYZ" score is high then the lesion is more likely to be a malignant melanoma [1–4].

The delay in detection of skin cancer may also lead to death in case of People of Color (PoC) who are less likely to be affected with skin cancer. Chronic stages of skin cancer are diagnosed in PoC which makes the treatment difficult. By improving the awareness regarding the color of the skin and its variation among the public, skin cancers can be detected at early stages and can also be cured. The data on various types of skin cancers were collected and presented to PoC. The detailed information about the dark-colored pigmented skin blisters is not available. Diagnostic features for different types of skin cancers were recorded and various possible risk factors were considered. As a result, a guideline was suggested to prevent and detect the skin cancers in PoC at early stages. Hence, it was concluded that the mortality rate can be decreased if the detection scheme is based on PoC. Raising public health awareness about skin cancer prevention strategies for all people, regardless of ethnic background and socioeconomic status, is the key to timely diagnosis and treatment [5–9].

Automated classification of skin lesions using images is a challenging task and it is carried out using SOM to classify the skin lesions. Performance of the algorithm is tested using binary classification of keratinocyte carcinomas versus benign seborrheic keratoses; and malignant melanomas versus benign [10–13].

Different algorithms are being introduced in the field of medical image processing that are based on the computational methods like image segmentation to diagnose the problems associated with different tissues and organs. The common and serious threat to people is cancer and the most common type of malignancy is the skin cancer. To provide solutions for such threats, researchers have invented robust and automated approaches like social group optimization (SGO) to examine skin melanoma. This algorithm uses Otsu/Kapur-based thresholding technique and active contour segmentation. The metrics like Jaccard's coefficient, Dice's coefficient, false positive/negative rate, accuracy, sensitivity, and specificity were used to validate the performance of the algorithm. Finally, it was inferred that SGO-based Kapur's thresholding technique with the level set-based segmentation technique served as a powerful tool for detecting melanoma from dermoscopy digital images with high sensitivity, specificity, and accuracy [14].

Skin melanoma has been proven to be the most fatal form of skin malignancies in human community. To offer an effective solution to the threat, an algorithm needs to be incorporated to support the clinical detection and diagnosis process. The two methods that are widely used to detect the skin cancers are visual inspection and the digital dermoscopy. Kapur's multithresholding and level set-based segmentation is used for detection of skin cancer. The experimental results state that the proposed method offers superior values of Jaccard (0.8805), Dice (0.9138), sensitivity (0.9927), specificity (0.9177), and accuracy (0.9628) [15].

The background behind this research work is to recognize and authorize a group of significant features to differentiate the benign from malignant lesions. The methods used comprise two datasets with 70 melanomas and 100 nevi, which contained raw images and also noise removal because of uneven illumination. The images were segmented and features like shape, color, asymmetry, eccentricity, circularity, asymmetry of color distribution, quadrant asymmetry, fast Fourier transform (FFT) normalization amplitude, and 6th and 7th Hu's moments were extracted. Feature selection was done using receiver operating characteristic (ROC) curve and area under the curve (AUC) to distinguish between nevi and melanoma. Accuracy is used as the performance measure for evaluating the efficiency of the proposed method [16].

Skin cancer is a malignancy which is primarily diagnosed visually, beginning with an initial clinical screening and followed potentially by dermoscopic analysis, a biopsy, and a histopathological examination [17–21].

2.4 METHODOLOGY

The images of the skin with noncancerous and highly cancerous skin sores are considered for this diagnosis. Images with sores on the skin are taken from the DermIS (http://www.dermis.net) and DermQuest (http://www.dermquest.com) databases. The sample dataset is illustrated in Table 2.1. This database consists of images which comprise nearly 281 noncancerous and 281 highly cancerous images of skin blisters. The procedural schematic for diagnosis of skin cancer is highlighted in Figure 2.3.

The various feature extraction techniques are discussed in the following subsections to enable the readers to have a thorough understanding of the techniques used. It comprises extraction methods for LBP features, Variance, Discrete Fourier Transform (DFT) coefficients, and their additive fused coefficients.

2.4.1 Computation of Local Binary Pattern (LBP)

In addition to the learning algorithm for computing the LBP features, the readers must have knowledge about the importance of LBP features, mathematics behind LBP features and also the corresponding algorithm.

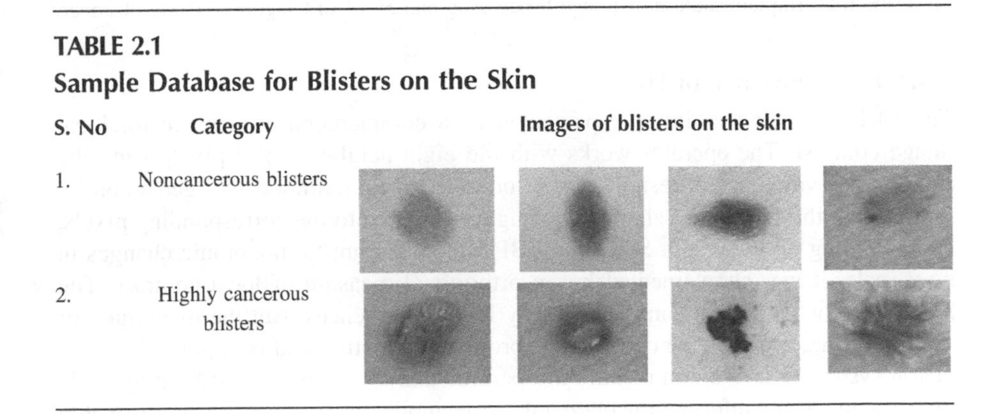

TABLE 2.1
Sample Database for Blisters on the Skin

S. No	Category	Images of blisters on the skin
1.	Noncancerous blisters	
2.	Highly cancerous blisters	

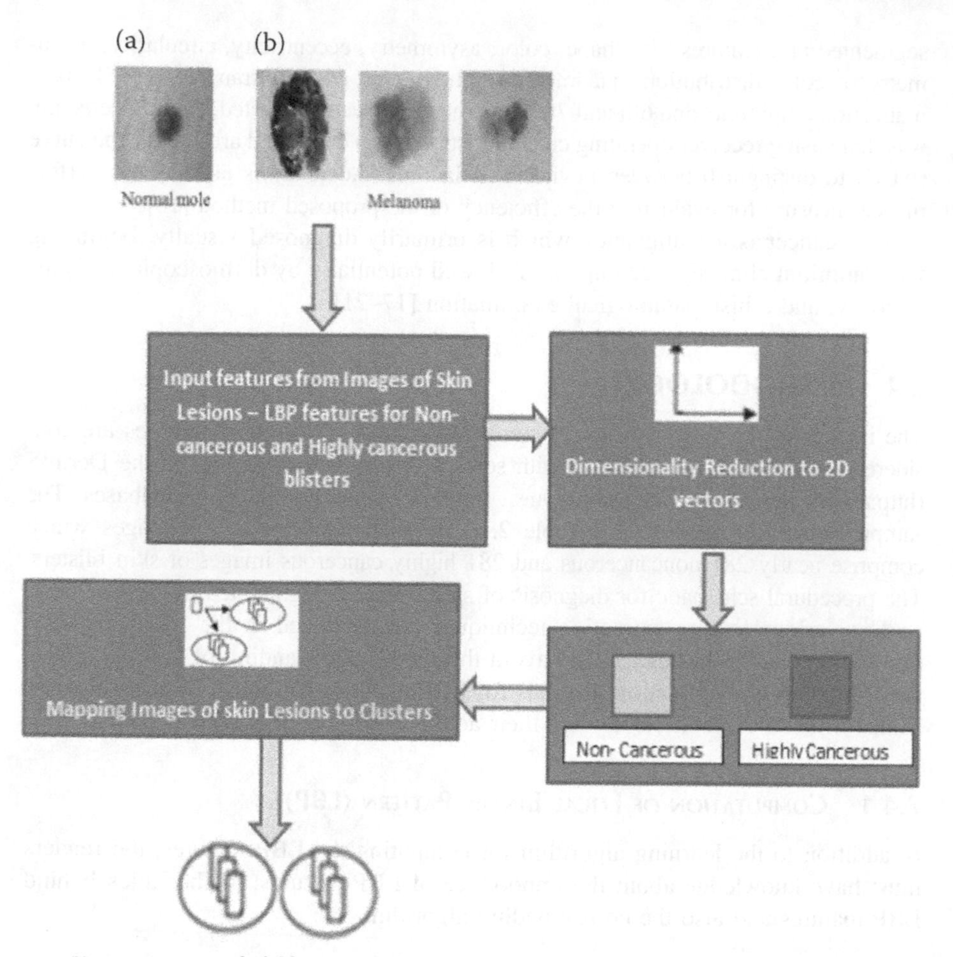

FIGURE 2.3 Implementation of Image Processing and SOM in Diagnosis of Skin Cancer.

2.4.1.1 Importance of LBP

The LBP operator was initially presented as a complementary measure for local image contrast. The operator works with the eight neighbors of a pixel, using the center pixel value as a threshold. LBP code for a neighborhood was generated by multiplying the threshold values with weights assigned to the corresponding pixels, and summing up the result. Since the LBP was, invariant to monotonic changes in gray scale, it was supplemented by an orthogonal measure of local contrast. The LBP operator ignores the amount of gray level divergences. But the magnitude of gray level that provides the contrast is a property of texture and is important for our vision system to arrive at a result. An operator that is not influenced by gray scale may waste useful information obtained from applications that have a reasonable control on illumination accurately. The accuracy of the operator can be enhanced by including information about gray scale. Texture is identified with two properties – spatial structure and contrast. Spatial structure is independent on gray scale and affected by rotation whereas contrast is dependent on gray scale but not affected by rotation. A joint distribution of LBP operator and local contrast measure as a texture descriptor will serve as a useful feature set. An operator formed with joint distribution of LBP and local variance can be formed. The texture descriptor thus formed will not vary with rotation. Basically, the derivation for LBP operator is discussed in Section 2.4.2.

2.4.2 Derivation for LBP

The mathematics behind LBP feature extraction is highlighted in this section. The texture "*T*" in a local neighborhood of a gray scale image is defined as the joint distribution of the gray levels of $P + 1$ ($P > 0$) image pixels as in Equation 2.1

$$T = t\,(g_c, g_0 \cdots \cdots, g_{p-1}) \tag{2.1}$$

where g_c corresponds to the gray value of the center pixel of a local neighborhood. g_p ($p = 0, 1, 2, 3 \ldots \ldots, P - 1$) corresponds to the gray values of 'P' pixels equally spaced on a circle of radius R ($R > 0$) that form a circularly symmetric set of neighbors. This set of $P + 1$ pixels is later denoted by 'G_P'. In a digital image domain, the coordinates of the g_P neighbors are given by $(x_c + R\cos(2\Pi p/P),\ y_c - R\sin(2\Pi p/P))$ where (x_c, y_c) are the coordinates of the center pixel.

The values of neighbors that do not fall exactly on pixels are estimated by bilinear interpolation and the operator can be expressed using Equation 2.2

$$T = t\,(g_c, g_0 - g_c \cdots \cdots, g_{p-1} - g_c) \tag{2.2}$$

Assuming that the differences are independent of g_c, the distribution can be factorized as in Equation 2.3:

$$T \approx t\,(g_c),\ t\,(g_0 - g_c \cdots \cdots, g_{p-1} - g_c) \tag{2.3}$$

Since $t\,(g_c)$ describes the overall luminance of an image, which is unrelated to local image texture, it does not provide useful information for texture analysis. Equation 2.4 simplifies to

$$T \approx t\,(g_0 - g_c \cdots \cdots, g_{p-1} - g_c) \tag{2.4}$$

The P-dimensional difference distribution records the occurrences of different texture patterns in the neighborhood of each pixel. For constant or slowly varying regions, the differences cluster near zero. On a spot, all differences are relatively large. On an edge, differences in some directions are larger than the others. Although invariant against gray scale shifts, the differences are affected by scaling. To achieve invariance with respect to any monotonic transformation of the gray scale, only the signs of the differences are considered as in Equations 2.5 and 2.6, respectively

$$T \approx t\left(s(g_0 - g_c) \ldots \ldots, s(g_{p-1} - g_c)\right) \tag{2.5}$$

where

$$s(x) = \begin{cases} 1 & s \geq 0 \\ 0 & s < 0 \end{cases} \tag{2.6}$$

Now, a binomial weight 2^p is assigned to each sign $s(g_p - g_c)$, transforming the differences in a neighborhood into a unique LBP code. The code characterizes the local image texture around (x_c, y_c)

$$LBP_{P,R}(x_c, y_c) = \sum_{p}^{P-1} s(g_p - g_c)2^p \tag{2.7}$$

In practice, Equation 2.7 means the signs of the differences in a neighborhood. The local gray scale distribution is denoted in Equation 2.8

$$T \approx t\left(LBP_{P,R}(x_c, y_c)\right) \tag{2.8}$$

Take $N \times M$ image with ($x_c \in \{0, 1, 2, \ldots., N - 1\}$, $y_c \in \{0, 1, 2 \ldots., M - 1\}$). The pixel at the center is considered for neighborhood calculation so that there are many pixel values available satisfying the adjacency condition rather than in the boundary region. The LBP code is calculated is denoted by S in Equation 2.9

$$S = t\left(LBR_{P,R}(x, y)\right) \tag{2.9}$$

where $x \in \{[R], \ldots \ldots, N - 1 - [R]\}$, $y \in \{[R], \ldots \ldots, M - 1 - [R]\}$.

The section below throws light about the algorithm for computation of LBP features to the readers.

2.4.3 Algorithm for LBP

The step-by-step procedure for computation of LBP features is indicated below.

- Split the inspected skin image into cells (e.g., $n \times n$ pixels for each cell).
- For every pixel in a cell, match the pixel to its every neighbor. Track the pixels in a circular form in clockwise or anticlockwise direction.
- Assume a threshold which states that the value of the pixel at the center is greater than the neighbor's value, and then make the answer as "0."

- Else, make the answer as "1." This yields a binary number which is typically transformed to a decimal value.

The purpose of experiments is to estimate and prove the capability of the LBP operator to represent the medical images mathematically. Experiments are performed separately to test the capacity of the operator so as to cluster the images and to retrieve them.

2.5 IMPORTANCE AND ALGORITHM FOR COMPUTATION OF VARIANCE

Statistics is a branch that deals with gathering, organizing, analyzing, and understanding the data. It handles all phases, which includes the plan to collect the data that would assist the design of survey and experimentation results. The different statistical measures include mean, deviation, variance, and standard deviation. All these measures are widespread and cater to the needs of technical and societal investigation, comprising various fields of studies.

- Read skin images
- Compute mean of the intensities in each image
- Determine the Deviation = Reference Image – Mean
- Calculate the Standard Deviation = Current Image – Deviation Value
- Infer Variance = (Standard Deviation)^2
- Repeat the above steps for all the images until the variance is computed for total images

2.6 ALGORITHM FOR DFT COMPUTATION

DFT refers to the frequency content of a digital signal with which operations like addition and power spectrum computation can be performed. It represents the comparable frequency domain characteristics. It is capable of approximating the coefficients of continuous Fourier transform. DFT is capable of providing an efficient approximation when sampling is carried out at Nyquist rate. If the Nyquist rate is violated then aliasing takes place, which affects the quality of the images. The flowchart is depicted in Figure 2.4.

Thus, this basic retrieval system that classifies and retrieves images using LBP, with variance, additive fusion, and DFT coefficients (without help of a trained classifier) was tested and the results are shown in Table 2.2.

From Table 2.2, the following inference is drawn. Extraction of LBP, variance, and the additive fusion values from the highly cancerous and noncancerous skin lesions, clearly states that the complete information can be retrieved for developing an automated skin cancer detection system which is comparable with the equivalent "VXYZ" rule for "ABCDE" rule practiced by the dermatologists.

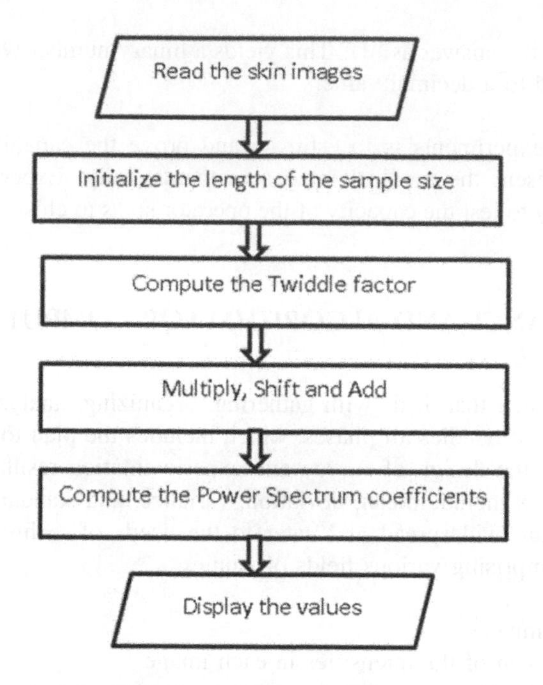

FIGURE 2.4 Flowchart for DFT Computation.

2.7 DETECTION OF SKIN LESION USING SELF-ORGANIZING MAPS (SOM)

The images of the skin with highly cancerous and noncancerous tumors are taken as inputs to the SOM. It is also called Kohonen neural network. It is an active tool for investigating the multiple dimension data. This neural network is incorporated for grouping the images of the skin with highly cancerous and noncancerous lesions, thereby preserving the feature of the image in such a way that related feature inputs stay at a minimum distance in the output layer of the network. SOM can robotically cluster distinct groups of images using an unsupervised technique.

This technique contains of three stages: at the first stage, a set of rules to infer "second winner" is implemented, in which the processing elements (PEs) in the competitive layer discover the initial position in the n-dimensional space. At the second stage, a technique named "batch learning" is engaged, and at the completion of this stage, training of the SOM is achieved. Last, at the third stage, data grouping is finished by eliminating the incorrect associations between the PEs. The features from two sets of images of skin lesions are deployed to demonstrate the accuracy and efficiency of the proposed method. Thereafter a weight matrix is defined with LBP as the input features from the skin lesion images without loss of information about the spatial distribution. The weight matrix performs the work of a filter removing the unwanted information and restoring the significant information from the original skin image matrix. The weights acting like a filter help in extraction of the boundaries without color variation and blur.

TABLE 2.2
Group-Wise Sample Values for DFT Coefficients, LBP, Variance, and Additive Fusion for Retrieval of Images with Skin Cancer

Training				Testing			
LBP values	Variance	Additive fusion	DFT coefficients	LBP values	Variance	Additive fusion	DFT coefficients
54.10	36.50	90.6	0.0002	38.89	41.86	80.75	0.0044
58.00	39.02	97.02	0.0003	36.11	55.81	91.92	0.0026
48.00	46.34	94.34	0.0015	38.89	48.83	87.72	0.0031
58.00	41.46	99.46	0.0029	41.66	44.18	85.84	0.0058
54.00	36.58	90.58	0.0026	36.11	37.20	73.31	0.0052
52.50	36.58	89.08	0.0028	38.88	34.88	73.76	0.0056
68.00	53.66	121.66	0.0046	58.33	53.49	111.82	0.0092
72.00	63.41	135.41	0.0009	63.89	55.14	119.03	0.0018
68.00	60.98	128.98	0.0005	61.11	51.16	112.27	0.0012
62.00	46.34	108.34	0.0011	47.22	48.84	96.06	0.0022
54.00	43.90	97.9	0.0006	44.44	46.51	90.95	0.0042
62.00	58.54	120.54	0.0020	58.33	51.16	109.49	0.0024
55.35	48.78	104.13	0.0012	52.78	48.83	101.61	0.0024
62.00	51.21	113.21	0.0005	50.00	44.18	94.18	0.0025
60.00	48.78	108.78	0.0007	55.00	44.18	99.18	0.0049
70.00	63.41	133.41	0.0006	63.89	51.16	115.05	0.0036
64.00	51.21	115.21	0.0032	58.33	51.16	109.49	0.0064
58.00	48.78	106.78	0.0036	47.22	44.18	91.4	0.0072
68.00	58.54	126.54	0.0049	63.89	48.84	112.73	0.0098
62.00	43.90	105.9	0.0023	44.44	55.81	100.25	0.0046
60.00	48.78	108.78	0.0007	52.77	48.83	101.6	0.0014

A "self-organizing map" (SOM) is a kind of Artificial Neural Network (ANN) that is accomplished using unsupervised learning technique to produce a two dimensional information, in the form of discrete data illustration on the input space during training of sample images, called a "map," and so this method reduces the dimension during mapping. SOM varies from other types of ANN because SOM uses competitive learning technique as conflicting to the adjustment of deviation like the back propagation algorithm with steepest gradient descent rule, and is dependent on the neighborhood function to conserve the topology of the input feature vector.

Every single point corresponding to the pixel in the input dataset is identified by competing for illustration. SOM mapping begins with initialization of the values for connection strengths. From this point the input samples are designated in an ad hoc fashion to form a map with the connection strengths explored to discover the optimal set of weights representing the input vectors. Every vector corresponding to the weight has adjacent weights which are adjacent to it. The selected weights are compensated and are randomly selected for a trial. The adjacent values to that of the weights are also compensated to be the selected sample vector. Hence, permission is granted for development of a map, which acquires various forms. Mostly, it can take any geometrical shape like square or rectangle or hexagon in 2D feature space.

The flow chart for the SOM algorithm is illustrated in Figure 2.5.

1. Initialize the connection strength (weight) values at every PE.
2. Identify a random input from the training set.
3. At each node the similarity is computed to find a suitable match with that of the input vector. Thus, the winning node is determined and is called as the Superlative Matching Unit (SMU).
4. Then the neighborhood of the SMU is inferred. The quantity of neighbors reduces after some time.
5. The winning weight is remunerated by becoming the sample vector. Their neighbors also become more like the sample vector. The nearer a node to the SMU, the more its weights get changed and the farer away the node is from the neighborhood of the SMU, the slower is the rate of learning.
6. Repeat step 2 for "N" number of iterations.
7. SMU is the method which computes the distance measure from each weight value to the sample vector, by scanning all weight vectors. The weight with the minimum distance is the winner. There are many ways to regulate the distance measure and one such method is the L1 or Manhattan distance measure, Euclidean distance measure or L2, d1 distance measure, and Canberra distance measures are used for implementation.

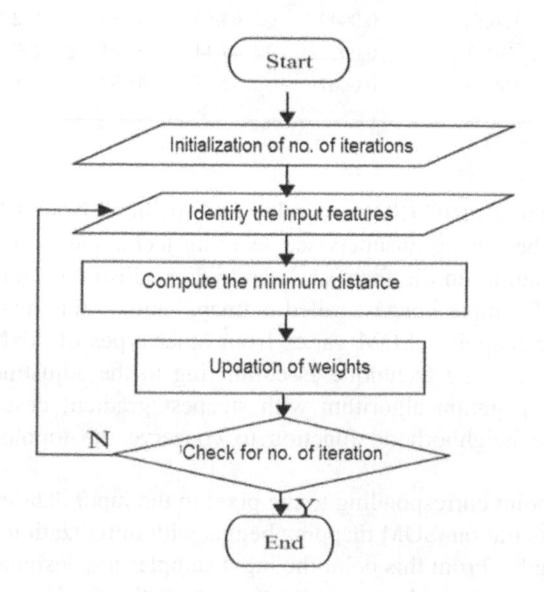

FIGURE 2.5 Flowchart for SOM.

If the mean distance exceeds a threshold, then the neighboring weights are dissimilar and that those images are clustered to benign skin lesion category. If the mean distance is less than a threshold, then the neighboring weights of those images are clustered to malignant skin lesion category. Therefore, the finalized weights will now be capable of extracting useful information for the input feature set presented to the SOM from the original skin image with lesions so that this value of error will help in accurate diagnosis of benign and malignant skin tumors. Figure 2.6 depicts the output for SOM in categorizing the skin images as highly cancerous and noncancerous skin lesions during training process. The output for identification efficacy (IE) of highly cancerous and noncancerous skin lesions by SOM is illustrated in Figure 2.7 for testing.

2.8 SIMILARITY MEASURES USED FOR TRAINING THE SOM

The objective of any CBIR system is to retrieve the highly cancerous and noncancerous skin images from an image database that resemble the reference image with skin lesions in each category. The selection of images that gives an optimal match is selected by measuring the minimum distance between the reference image and the other images in the database. In this implementation, four types of similarity distance metrics have been used for the purpose of determining the optimally closest match which is expressed in Equation 2.10 to Equation 2.13, respectively.

L_1 or Manhattan distance measure or city block distance measure

$$D(Q, DB_j) = \sum_{i=1}^{lf} |(f_{DBji} - f_{Qi})| \tag{2.10}$$

L_2 or Euclidean distance measure:

$$D(Q, DB_j) = \sqrt{\sum_{i=1}^{lf} (f_{DBji} - f_{Qi})^2} \tag{2.11}$$

Canberra distance measure:

$$D(Q, DB_j) = \sum_{i=1}^{lf} \frac{|(f_{DBji} - f_{Qi})|}{|f_{DBji}| + |f_{Qi}|} \tag{2.12}$$

d_1 distance measure:

$$D(Q, DB_j) = \sum_{i=1}^{lf} \left| \frac{(f_{DBji} - f_{Qi})}{1 + f_{DBji} + f_{Qi}} \right| \tag{2.13}$$

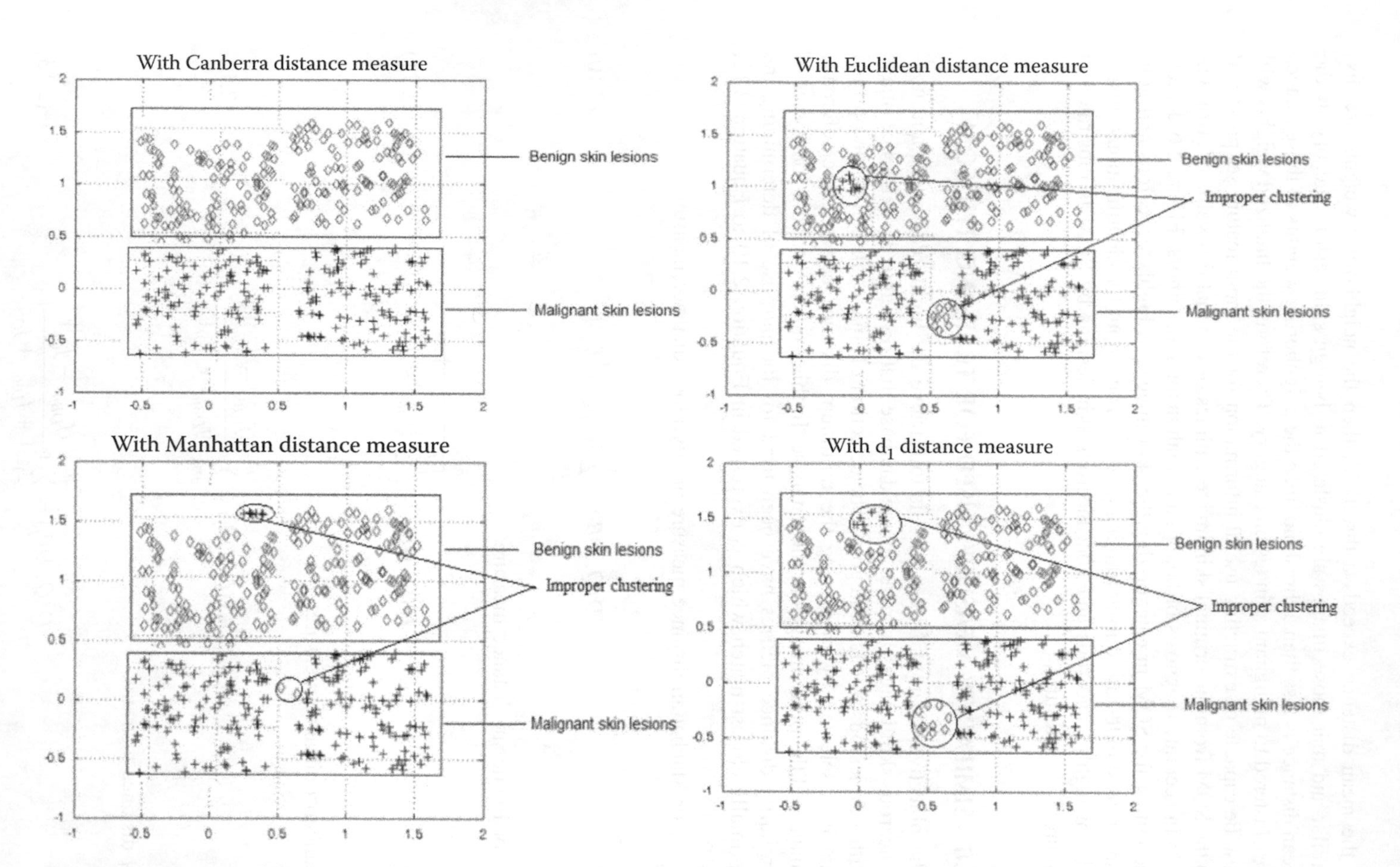

FIGURE 2.6 Identification of Highly Cancerous and Noncancerous Skin Lesions by SOM Training.

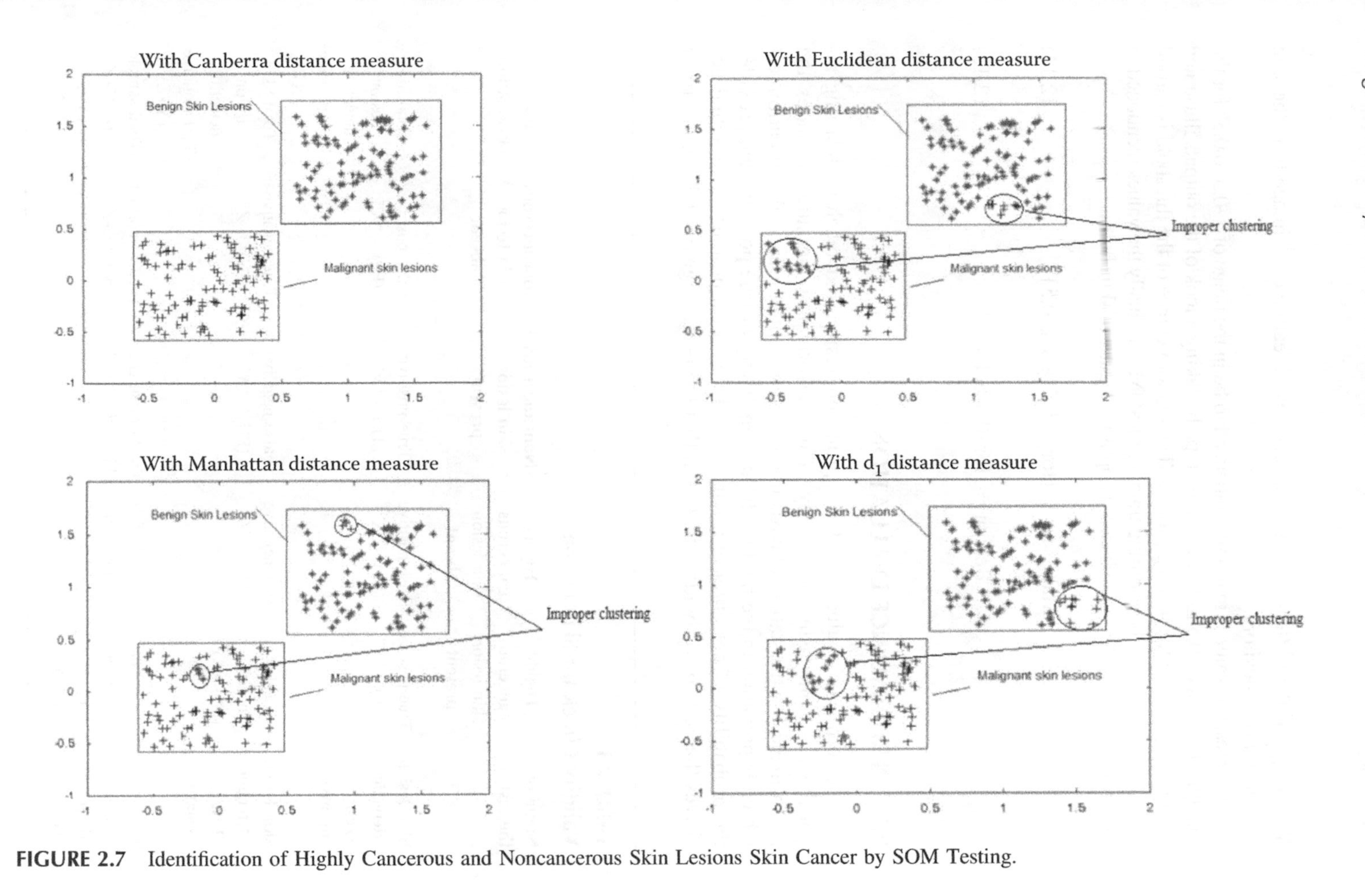

FIGURE 2.7 Identification of Highly Cancerous and Noncancerous Skin Lesions Skin Cancer by SOM Testing.

Where f_{DBji} is the jth (length of feature vector is l_f) feature of ith image from the skin cancer image repository.

The threshold value is randomly initialized to be in the range of "–0.5 to 0.5" for the malignant type and "0.5 to 1" for benign type by taking a look of the outputs illustrated in Figure 2.5 during the training process. The random choice of the threshold is carried out on a trial and error basis during training of SOM and finally the values mentioned in Equations 2.14 and 2.15 are chosen as optimal values of threshold.

$$\text{Malignant} = \{\text{for} - 0.5 \geq \text{T} \geq 0.5\} \tag{2.14}$$

$$\text{Benign} = \{\text{for } 0.5 \geq \text{T} \geq 1\} \tag{2.15}$$

2.9 PERFORMANCE EVALUATION

The performance evaluation of the proposed vision and machine learning algorithms is done using sensitivity. This performance measure evaluates the performance on the statistical basis using the concept of binary classification test which is prevalent in the medical field. Sensitivity or true positive rate provides the probability of detection in the medicinal field as a proportion of actual positives that are correctly identified such that the percentage of highly cancerous/

TABLE 2.3
Validity Check for Skin Lesion

Name of the test	Highly cancerous skin lesion present	Highly cancerous skin lesion absent	Noncancerous skin lesion present	Noncancerous skin lesion absent	Total test evaluation
Skin lesion detection Test positive	True positive (TP) – "V"	False positive (FP) – "X"	True positive (TP) – "V"	False positive (FP) – "X"	Total Skin lesion detection Test positive (V+X)
Skin lesion detection Test negative	False negative (FN) – "Y"	True negative (TN) – "Z"	False negative (FN) – "Y"	True negative (TN) – "Z"	Total Skin lesion detection Test negative (Y+Z)
Total skin lesion detection Test	Total of malignant skin lesion (V+Y)	Total of normal skin (X+Z)	Total of malignant skin lesion (V+Y)	Total of normal skin (X+Z)	Total sample size V+X +Y+Z

noncancerous skin lesions which are correctly identified as highly cancerous and noncancerous skin lesions. The reference table for validity check is depicted in Table 2.3.

The cell "V" denotes the test in which the presence of highly cancerous/noncancerous skin lesion is correctly diagnosed. In other words, the skin lesion test is positive and algorithmic detection is also positive, which is called as True Positive (TP).

The cell "X" denotes the test in which positive results are obtained for malignant/benign skin lesion but does not have the malignant/benign lesion. The algorithmic detection is wrongly diagnosed as skin lesion and is called as False Positive (FP).

The cell "Y" denotes the skin lesion test which yields negative result by algorithmic detection but the lesion actually presents highly cancerous/noncancerous skin lesions. The skin lesion test has wrongly labeled a malignant/benign skin lesion "normal" and hence is called False Negative (FN).

The cell "Z" denotes the test that detects presence of normal skin by both the skin lesion test and algorithm, that is, negative, and hence is called True Negative (TN). Sensitivity is the ability of a test to correctly classify the presence of skin lesion as mentioned in Table 2.4(a). Similarly, the calculation for sensitivity analysis is depicted in Table 2.4(b). It is inferred that the sensitivity is in the range of "0.96 to 1" if Canberra and Manhattan distance measures are used for similarity check for training and testing the SOM.

2.10 RESULTS AND DISCUSSION

The automated skin cancer detection system using image processing techniques and deep learning algorithms serves as a major contribution in the field of medicine allowing radiologists to offer accurate diagnosis without manual error, so that an

TABLE 2.4(A)
Sensitivity Analysis

Name of the test	Highly cancerous skin blister present	Highly cancerous skin blister absent	Noncancerous skin blister present	Noncancerous skin blister absent
Skin blister detection Test positive	True positive (TP) – "V"	False positive (FP) – "X"	True positive (TP) – "V"	False positive (FP) – "X"
Skin blister detection Test negative	False negative (FN) – "Y"	True negative (TN) – "Z"	False negative (FN) – "Y"	True negative (TN) – "Z"
Sensitivity	V/(V+Y)		X/(X+Z)	

TABLE 2.4(B)
Calculation Matrix for Sensitivity Analysis

Name of the test	Detection phase	Highly cancerous skin blister present	Highly cancerous skin blister absent	Noncancerous skin blister present	Noncancerous skin blister absent
Skin blister detection Test positive		True positive (TP) – "V"	False positive (FP) – "X"	True positive (TP) – "V"	False positive (FP) – "X"
Skin blister detection Test positive – Canberra distance measure	Training Testing	198 78	1 1	198 78	1 1
Skin blister detection Test positive – Euclidean distance measure	Training Testing	192 75	7 5	192 69	7 11
Skin blister detection Test positive – Manhattan distance measure	Training Testing	195 77	4 3	198 77	1 3
Skin blister detection Test positive – $d_1$distance measure	Training Testing	190 71	9 9	190 71	9 9
Skin blister detection Test negative		False negative (FN) – "Y"	True negative (TN) – "Z"	False negative (FN) – "Y"	True negative (TN) – "Z"
Skin blister detection Test negative – Canberra distance measure	Training Testing	1 1	0 0	1 1	0 0
Skin blister detection Test negative – Euclidean distance measure	Training Testing	7 5	0 0	7 11	0 0
Skin blister detection Test negative –	Training Testing	4 3	0 0	1 3	0 0

TABLE 2.4(B) (Continued)
Calculation Matrix for Sensitivity Analysis

Name of the test	Detection phase	Highly cancerous skin blister present	Highly cancerous skin blister absent	Noncancerous skin blister present	Noncancerous skin blister absent
Manhattan distance measure					
Skin blister detection	Training	9	0	9	0
Test negative – $d_1$distance measure	Testing	9	0	9	0
Sensitivity		V/(V+Y)		X/(X+Z)	
Sensitivity for Canberra distance measure	Training	198/(198+1) = 0.99		1/(1+0) = 1	
	Testing	78/(78+1) = 0.98		1/(1+0) = 1	
Sensitivity for Euclidean distance measure	Training	192/(192+7) = 0.97		1/(1+0) = 1	
	Testing	75/(75+5) = 0.94		1/(1+0) = 1	
Sensitivity for Manhattan distance measure	Training	195/(195+4) = 0.98		1/(1+0) = 1	
	Testing	77/(77+3) = 0.96		1/(1+0) = 1	
Sensitivity for d_1 distance measure	Training	190/(190+9) = 0.95		1/(1+0) = 1	
	Testing	71/(71+9) = 0.88		1/(1+0) = 1	

appropriate treatment can be provided to the patients, thereby curing the disease at the right time without many complications.

The melanoma images are taken from the DermIS (http://www.dermis.net) and DermQuest (http://www.dermquest.com) databases. This database consists of nearly 281 benign and 281 images of malignant lesions. The SOM architecture for identification of highly cancerous and noncancerous skin lesions includes four neurons in the input layer with two neurons in the output layer which is the competitive layer. The four inputs to the SOM are LBP, variance, fused coefficients, and DFT coefficients, respectively. The two outputs in the competitive layer include the highly cancerous and noncancerous skin lesions. These images are preprocessed for noise and blur removal using Wiener filter so that the images with skin cancer can be restored and used for further error-free analysis. The LBP values, variance, and the additive fusion coefficients are used as inputs to train the SOM. The IE is tabulated in Table 2.5 which states that when Canberra and Manhattan distance measures are used, the clustering efficacy is high for identification of highly cancerous and noncancerous skin lesions.

TABLE 2.5
IE for Skin Cancer

S. no	Training/ Testing	Total no. of images with skin lesion		No. of images correctly identified skin lesion		% IE		Distance measure for SOM
		Noncancerous	Highly cancerous	Noncancerous	Highly cancerous	Non-cancerous	Highly cancerous	Type of distance measure
1.	Training	200	200	199	199	99.5	99.5	Canberra distance measure
	Testing	81	81	79	80	97.53	98.7	
2.	Training	200	200	192	192	96.2	96.2	Euclidean distance measure
	Testing	81	81	75	69	92.5	85.1	
3.	Training	200	200	195	198	97.5	99	Manhattan distance measure
	Testing	81	81	77	77	95.06	95.06	
4.	Training	200	200	190	190	95	95	d_1 distance measure
	Testing	81	81	71	71	87.6	87.6	

The proposed method is also validated by calculating the sensitivity of SOM algorithm in diagnosing skin cancer efficiently and is interpreted in Table 2.6(a) and (b). The percentage sensitivity for Test positive is calculated using the formula [V/(V+Y)] × 100% and for Test negative is found using [Y/(V+Y)] × 100%. Similarly, Test positive is defined as a test result that indicates whether a patient is diseased with either highly cancerous or noncancerous lesions on the skin. On the other hand, Test negative denotes that a test result indicates that these lesions on the skin are not malignant or benign lesions. The test positive results are in the range of 85% to 99% depending on the distance measure adopted for clustering the images with skin lesions by SOM. Likewise, the test negative results are in the range of 0.5% to 12% depending on the distance measure adopted for clustering the images with skin lesions by SOM. Canberra distance measure and Manhattan distance measure are almost similar types of distance measures which depend on computation of absolute difference. The reason is that the distinction is the absolute difference between the variables of the two categories, namely highly cancerous and noncancerous skin lesions, divided by the sum of the absolute variable values prior to summing. It is evident from Table 2.6(b) that the Canberra distance measure and Manhattan distance measure used in the competitive layer

TABLE 2.6(A)
Categorization by Various Distance Measures for Detection of Highly Cancerous/Noncancerous Skin Lesions

Distance measure in the competitive layer of SOM	Detection phase	Highly cancerous skin lesion present		Highly cancerous skin lesion absent		Noncancerous skin lesion present		Noncancerous skin lesion absent	
		TP (V)	FN (Y)	TN (Z)	FP (X)	TP (V)	FN (Y)	TN (Z)	FP (X)
Canberra distance measure	Training	198	1	0	1	198	1	0	1
	Testing	78	1	0	1	79	1	0	1
Euclidean distance measure	Training	192	7	0	1	192	7	0	1
	Testing	75	5	0	1	69	11	0	1
Manhattan distance measure	Training	195	4	0	1	198	1	0	1
	Testing	77	3	0	1	77	3	0	1
d_1 distance measure	Training	190	9	0	1	190	9	0	1
	Testing	71	9	0	1	71	9	0	1

TABLE 2.6(B)
Calculation for Sensitivity in Categorizing and Detection of Highly Cancerous/Noncancerous Skin Lesions

Name of the test	Detection phase	Highly cancerous skin lesion present	Highly cancerous skin lesion absent	Noncancerous skin lesion present	Noncancerous skin lesion absent
Sensitivity calculation for Test positive by Canberra distance measure	Training	V/(V+Y) = 198/(198+1)	X/(X+Z) = 1/(1+0)	V/(V+Y) = 198/(198+1)	X/(X+Z) = 1/(1+0)
	Testing	V/(V+Y) = 78/(78+1)	X/(X+Z) = 1/(1+0)	V/(V+Y) = 78/(78+1)	X/(X+Z) = 1/(1+0)
% Sensitivity for Test positive by Canberra distance measure	Training	99.5%	100%	99.5%	100%
	Testing	98.7%	100%	98.7%	100%
Sensitivity calculation for Test positive by Euclidean distance measure	Training	V/(V+Y) = 192/(192+7)	X/(X+Z) = 1/(1+0)	V/(V+Y) = 192/(192+7)	X/(X+Z) = 1/(1+0)
	Testing	V/(V+Y) = 75/(75+5)	X/(X+Z) = 1/(1+0)	V/(V+Y) = 69/(69+11)	X/(X+Z) = 1/(1+0)
% Sensitivity for Test positive by Euclidean distance measure	Training	96.4%	100%	96.4%	100%
	Testing	93.75%	100%	86.25%	100%
Sensitivity calculation for Test positive by Manhattan distance measure	Training	V/(V+Y) = 195/(195+4)	X/(X+Z) = 1/(1+0)	V/(V+Y) = 198/(198+1)	X/(X+Z) = 1/(1+0)
	Testing	V/(V+Y) = 77/(77+3)	X/(X+Z) = 1/(1+0)	V/(V+Y) = 77/(77+3)	X/(X+Z) = 1/(1+0)
% Sensitivity for Test positive by Manhattan distance measure	Training	97.98%	100%	99.4%	100%
	Testing	96.25%	100%	96.25%	100%
Sensitivity calculation for Test positive by $d_1$distance measure	Training	V/(V+Y) = 190/(190+9)	X/(X+Z) = 1/(1+0)	V/(V+Y) = 190/(190+9)	X/(X+Z) = 1/(1+0)
	Testing	V/(V+Y) = 71/(71+9)	X/(X+Z) = 1/(1+0)	V/(V+Y) = 71/(71+9)	X/(X+Z) = 1/(1+0)
% Sensitivity for Test positive by	Training	95.4%	100%	95.4%	100%

TABLE 2.6(B) (Continued)
Calculation for Sensitivity in Categorizing and Detection of Highly Cancerous/Noncancerous Skin Lesions

Name of the test	Detection phase	Highly cancerous skin lesion present	Highly cancerous skin lesion absent	Noncancerous skin lesion present	Noncancerous skin lesion absent
$d_1$distance measure	Testing	88.75%	100%	88.75%	100%
Sensitivity calculation for Test negative by Canberra distance measure	Training	Y/(V+Y) = 1/(198+1)	Z/(X+Z) = 0/(1+0)	Y/(V+Y) = 1/(198+1)	Z/(X+Z) = 0/ (1+0) = 0
	Testing	Y/(V+Y) = 1/(78+1)	Z/(X+Z) = 0/(1+0)	Y/(V+Y) = 1/(78+1)	Z/(X+Z) = 0/(1+0)
% Sensitivity for Test negative by Canberra distance measure	Training	0.5%	0%	0.5%	0%
	Testing	1.26%	0%	1.26%	0%
Sensitivity calculation for Test negative by Euclidean distance measure	Training	Y/(V+Y) = 7/(192+7)	Z/(X+Z) = 0(1+0) = 0	Y/(V+Y) =7/(192+7)	Z/(X+Z) = 0(1+0)
	Testing	Y/(V+Y) = 5/(5+75)	Z/(X+Z) = 0/(1+0)	Y/(V+Y) =11/(69+11)	Z/(X+Z) = 0/(1+0)
% Sensitivity for Test negative by Euclidean distance measure	Training	3.51%	0%	3.51%	0%
	Testing	6.25%	0%	13.75%	0%
Sensitivity calculation for Test negative by Manhattan distance measure	Training	Y/(V+Y) = 4/(195+4)	Z/(X+Z) = 0/(1+0)	Y/(V+Y) = 1/(198+1)	Z/(X+Z) = 0/(1+0)
	Testing	Y/(V+Y) = 4/(77+4)	Z/(X+Z) = 0/(1+0)	Y/(V+Y) = 4/(77+4)	Z/(X+Z) = 0/(1+0)
% Sensitivity for Test negative by Manhattan distance measure	Training	2.01%	0%	5.02%	0%
	Testing	4.9%	0%	4.9%	0%
Sensitivity calculation for Test negative by	Training	Y/(V+Y) = 9/(190+9)	Z/(X+Z) = 0(1+0)	Y/(V+Y) = 9/(190+9)	Z/(X+Z) = 0(1+0)
	Testing				Z/(X+Z)= 0/(1+0)

(Continued)

TABLE 2.6(B) (Continued)
Calculation for Sensitivity in Categorizing and Detection of Highly Cancerous/Noncancerous Skin Lesions

Name of the test	Detection phase	Highly cancerous skin lesion present	Highly cancerous skin lesion absent	Noncancerous skin lesion present	Noncancerous skin lesion absent
$d_1$distance measure		Y/(V+Y) = 9/(71+9)	Z/(X+Z) = 0/(1+0)	Y/(V+Y) = 9/(71+9)	
% Sensitivity for Test negative by $d_1$distance measure	Training	5%	0%	5%	0%
	Testing	11.25%	0%	11.25%	0%

for clustering the samples of the skin images based on the winner-take-all concept were able to identify the patterns with closest resemblance that too with an optimally smaller value of similarity index. It is also interpreted that the sensitivity values for the above said distance measures in competitive layer of the SOM was found to be 97% to 99%.

2.11 CONCLUSION

This chapter focuses on detecting skin cancer based on various features such as the power spectrum coefficient of DFT, LBP values, variance, and additive fusion of LBP and variance. The detection of highly cancerous and noncancerous skin lesions can be made using machine learning algorithms like SOM, in which the system is trained based on the history of the skin images stored in the database, and finds the closest match to the current skin image to determine whether the image under scrutiny is categorized to be highly cancerous or noncancerous at the initial stage itself. A comparison can be made with the various types of distance measures to find the optimal match (minimum distance) using SOM, which is a machine learning algorithm. Hence, the proposed algorithm reduces the computational complexity and the treatment can be carried out at the onset of lesion on the skin.

In this chapter, a novel vision machine technique has been proposed to diagnose the malignant/highly cancerous and benign/noncancerous skin lesions which are difficult for radiologists to identify manually at their early stage. Multiple image samples having benign and malignant lesions on the skin were used for this image-based diagnosis. Moreover, an optimal feature set is used for diagnosis of skin cancer. Skin lesion test as per the guidelines of the All India Medical Foundation is compared with the performance of the proposed image processing and machine learning methods. The test data has revealed that SOM was able to cluster the group of skin images using the DFT coefficients, LBP values, and variance features using additive fusion technique for training the model. The sensitivity is in the range of 85% to 99% and it effectively improves the IE of the integrated machine vision skin cancer detection system.

REFERENCES

[1]. Amelard, R., J. Glaister, A. Wong, and D. A. Clausi, "High-level intuitive features (HLIFs) for intuitive skin lesion description", *IEEE Transactions on Biomedical Engineering*, vol. 62, issue 3, pp. 820–831, October, 2015.

[2]. Glaister, J., R. Amelard, A. Wong, and D. A. Clausi, "MSIM: Multi-stage illumination modeling of dermatological photographs for illumination-corrected skin lesion analysis", *IEEE Transactions on Biomedical Engineering*, vol. 60, issue 7, pp. 1873–1883, November, 2013.

[3]. Chung, A., C. Scharfenberger, F. Khalvati, A. Wong, and M. A. Haider, "Statistical textural distinctiveness in multi-parametric prostate MRI for suspicious region detection", *International Conference on Image Analysis and Recognition (ICIAR)*, July, 2015.

[4]. Kazemzadeh, F., S. Haider, A. Wong, C. Scharfenberger, and D. A. Clausi, "Concurrent multiview discrete spectral imaging device from the VIS to the NIR", *SPIE: Optics + Photonics*, 2014.

[5]. Amelard, R., A. Wong, and D. A. Clausi, "Extracting morphological high-level intuitive features (HLIF) for enhancing skin lesion classification", *34th Annual International Conference of the IEEE Engineering in Medicine and Biology Society*, pp. 4458–4461, August, 2012.

[6]. Amelard, R., A. Wong, and D. A. Clausi, "Extracting high-level intuitive features (HLIF) for classifying skin lesions using standard camera images", *9th Conference on Computer and Robot Vision*, pp. 396–403, May, 2012.

[7]. Glaister, J., A. Wong, and D. A. Clausi, "Illumination correction in dermatological photographs using multi-stage illumination modeling for skin lesion analysis", *34th Annual International Conference of the IEEE Engineering in Medicine and Biology*, pp. 102–105, 2012.

[8]. Amelard, R., J. Glaister, A. Wong, and D. A. Clausi, "Melanoma decision support using lighting-corrected intuitive feature models", in *Computer vision techniques for the diagnosis of skin cancer*, pp. 193–219. Springer, Berlin, 2013.

[9]. Amelard, R., "High-level intuitive features (HLIFs) for melanoma detection", *Department of Systems Design Engineering*, pp. 85, 2013.

[10]. Glaister, J., "Automatic segmentation of skin lesions from dermatological photographs", *Department of Systems Engineering*, *University of Waterloo*, 2013.

[11]. LeCun, Y., Y. Bengio, and G. Hinton, "Deep learning". *Nature,* vol. 521, pp. 436–444, 2015.

[12]. LeCun, Y., and Y. Bengio, *The handbook of brain theory and neural networks* (ed.Arbib, M. A.), MIT Press, Cambridge, 1995.

[13]. Russakovsky, O. et al., "Imagenet large scale visual recognition challenge". *International Journal of Computer Vision,* vol. 115, pp. 211–252, 2015.

[14]. Dey, Nilanjan, Venkatesan Rajinikanth, Amira S. Ashour, and João Manuel R. S. Tavares, "Social group optimization supported segmentation and evaluation of skin melanoma images". *Symmetry*, vol. 10,issue 2, pp. 51, 2018.

[15]. Rajinikanth, Venkatesan, Suresh Chandra Satapathy, Nilanjan Dey, Steven Lawrence Fernandes, and K. Suresh Manic, "Skin melanoma assessment using

Kapur's entropy and level set—A study with bat algorithm", in *Smart intelligent computing and applications,* pp. 193–202. Springer, Singapore, 2019.

[16]. Damian, Felicia Anisoara, Simona Moldovanu, Nilanjan Dey, and Luminita Moraru, "Feature selection of non-dermoscopic skin lesion images for nevus and melanoma classification. Computation". *Symmetry*, vol. 8, issue 2, pp. 41, 2020.

[17]. Szegedy, C. et al., "Going deeper with convolutions", *IEEE Conference on Computer Vision and Pattern Recognition*, pp. 1–9, 2015.

[18]. He, K., X. Zhang, S. Ren, and J. Sun, "Deep residual learning for image recognition". 2015, preprint at https://arxiv.org/abs/1512.03385.

[19]. Masood, A., and A. A. Al-Jumaily, "Computer aided diagnostic support system for skin cancer: A review of techniques and algorithms". *International Journal of Biomedical Imaging,* vol. 2013, pp. 323268, 2013.

[20]. Cerwall, P., and E. M. Report, "Ericssons mobility report", *Ericsson.Com*, 2016, https://www.ericsson.com/res/docs/2016/ericsson-mobility-report-2016.pdf.

[21]. Rosado, B. et al., "Accuracy of computer diagnosis of melanoma: A quantitative meta-analysis". *Archives of Dermatology,* vol. 139, pp. 361–367, discussion 366, 2003.

3 Innovative Wearable Device Technology for Biomedical Applications

Arpan Ghosh[1,2], *Taranjeet Kaur*[3], *Pritam Dhalla*[2], *Aryan Jaiswal*[1,2], *Nirmal Kumar Mohakud*[4], *Santosh Kumar Panda*[4], *Namrata Misra*[1,2], *and Mrutyunjay Suar*[1,2]

[1]School of Biotechnology, Kalinga Institute of Industrial Technology, Deemed to be University (KIIT DU), Bhubaneswar, India

[2]KIIT Technology Business Incubator (KIIT-TBI), Kalinga Institute of Industrial Technology (KIIT-DU), Deemed to be University, Bhubaneswar, India

[3]Entrepreneurship Development and Strategic Partnership, Biotechnology Industry Research Assistance Council (BIRAC), New Delhi, India

[4]Department of Pediatrics, Kalinga Institute of Medical Sciences, KIIT Deemed to Be University, Bhubaneswar, India

CONTENTS

DOI: 10.1201/9781003198796-3

3.1 INTRODUCTION

The global healthcare system has witnessed several significant advancements and breakthroughs over the past few years, particularly with respect to improved life expectancy and better affordable treatment of various infectious diseases. In this regard, wearable technologies and medical devices are playing a strategic role by allowing early diagnosis of diseases and real-time monitoring of health parameters. Although there are varied definitions in scientific literature of "wearable devices," however, in simple terms, it is described as "devices that can be worn or coupled with human body to closely monitor an individual's activities and health continuously, without interrupting the user's motion" (Haghi et al., 2017).

Rapid increase in lifestyle-related diseases over the past few years has led to a higher demand for health monitoring wearable devices, which would continuously monitor and provide real-time updates on various health parameters like – heart rate, pulse, oxygen saturation, etc. to the user as well as to the clinicians (Hayward et al., 2017; Joshi et al., 2019). Some of these technologies are becoming part of our every day life in the form of smart watches, glasses, contact lenses, orthopedic shoes, and smart fabrics as they are convenient, portable, and mostly offer hands-free access to electronics. Advancements in electronic fabrication and packaging technologies have enabled integrating many microsensors onto medical devices at a very low cost. These improve their sensitivity and specificity for sensing of various vital parameters of the human body (Ozcan, 2014). The general architecture of wearables comprises four modules as shown in Figure 3.1 (Dias and Paulo Silva, 2018).

The Body Area Network comprises a network of sensors placed around the human body. The vital signs and other important information from these sensors are then transmitted to the portable unit which subsequently performs signal processing for extracting important features to evaluate the user health status. The raw data collected by the portable unit could be further transmitted using a wireless system for further use in clinical analysis or to maintain personal health record (Dias and Paulo Silva, 2018). With the integration of Internet of Things (IoT) in the wearable devices, the medical devices got the ability to continuously monitor different vital statistics of patients remotely at an affordable cost by using simple mobile network technologies, particularly for low resource-setting regions in a country (Koydemir and Ozcan, 2018; Vashist et al., 2014; Bhatt et al., 2017).

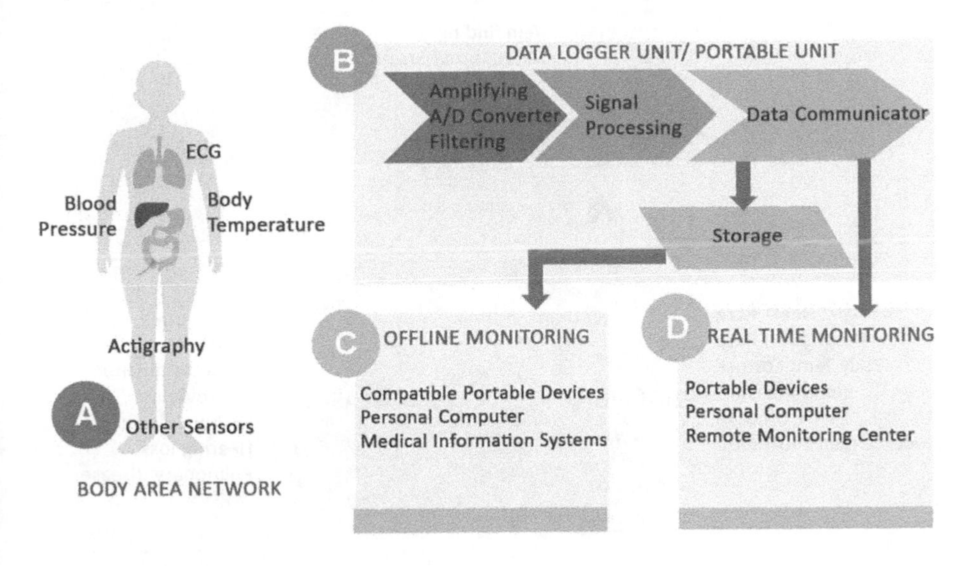

FIGURE 3.1 Framework of wearable medical devices system.

This chapter highlights the current scenario of wearable devices and sensors for healthcare applications. Specifically, it focuses on some widely used commercially available wearable devices for continuous gauging patient's vital parameters and discusses the major factors influencing the surge in the demand for medical devices. Furthermore, this chapter addresses the major factors that need to be considered in future through innovative approaches for widespread utilization of wearables in healthcare applications.

3.2 WEARABLE DEVICES IN VITAL SIGNS MONITORING

Recent advancements in sensor technologies and their varied applications have enabled the researchers in the healthcare domain to fabricate several varieties of wearable devices useful for vital signs monitoring and for various biomedical applications mentioned in Figure 3.2 (Koydemir and Ozcan, 2018). Currently, the wide range of wearable devices available in the market for monitoring several health parameters are smartphone-enabled, thereby allowing the user to interpret the data rapidly (Chan et al., 2012). In particular, heart rate, respiration rate, blood oxygen saturation level, body temperature, blood pressure, calories burnt, and blood glucose are the major vital signs widely examined continuously to identify clinical deterioration (Dias and Paulo Silva, 2018). Additionally, these devices also measure other parameters to understand the condition of the patient's health from daily activities, such as motion trackers (Haghi et al., 2018), calories burned, step monitoring, sleep patterns, and eating habits (Koydemir and Ozcan, 2018). This section discusses the various vital parameters that can be monitored using wearable body sensors.

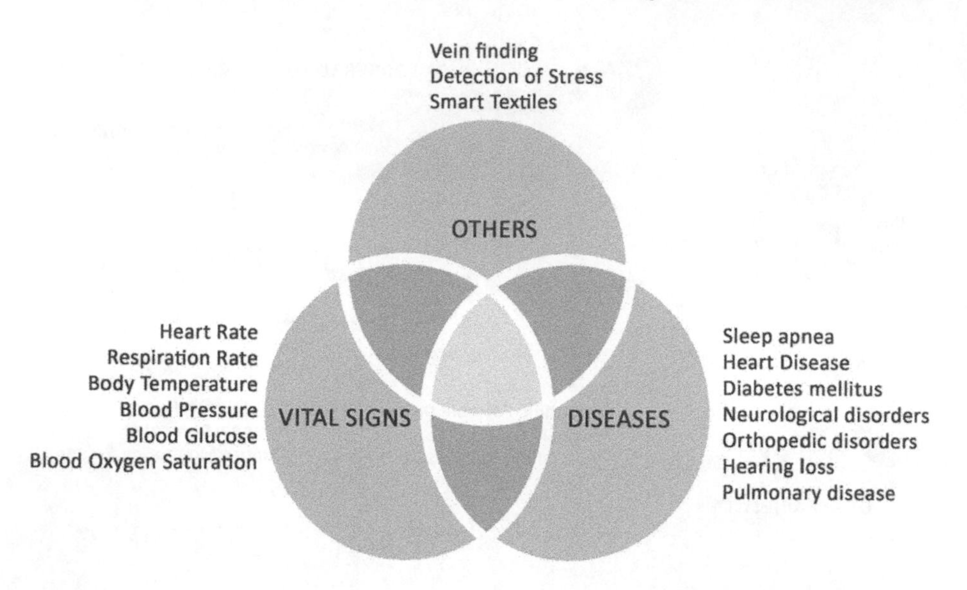

FIGURE 3.2 An overview of various applications of wearable health devices in healthcare.

3.2.1 Heart Rate

Heart rate is considered as the most frequently measured vital sign, specifically in both healthcare and fitness/sports fields to unravel the functioning of the heart during exercise (Koydemir and Ozcan, 2018). This vital sign is generally extracted from the ECG (R-peak) or photoplethysmography (PPG) signals. These signals are from different physiological origins and have different underpinning data in their wave forms, nevertheless, they contain alike heart rate information (Dey et al., 2017; Zhang et al., 2014). Besides these, many alternative methods are also present to determine heart rate, like using inertial sensors (Aarts et al., 2017) or scales (Giovangrandi et al., 2012), named Ballisto Cardiogram (BCG), however, these methods are not as reliable as compared to the heart rate interpreted from the ECG and PPG (Dias and Paulo Silva, 2018).

The first wearable wireless wristband was manufactured in the 1980s to observe the real-time heart rate of athletes during strenuous physical movements (Stahl et al., 2016). Currently, several wearable sensors are available in the market for providing real-time heart rate measurements, not only during strenuous activities like running, walking, or exercise but also at rest. Additionally, the devices can measure the heart rate from various body parts such as the ear, wrist, finger, and chest, through optical sensors, gyroscopes, accelerometers, and pressure sensors embedded in the wearables (Olmez and Dokur, 2003). A list of few commercially wearable devices for measuring heart rate is given in Table 3.1. Furthermore, these devices are also capable of providing the graphical interpretation of the data that the device has measured earlier together with the Global Positioning System (GPS) information for optimum performance study.

TABLE 3.1
Overview of Commercially Available Wearable Devices for Measurement of Heart Rate (Koydemir and Ozcan, 2018)

Wearable device	Body parts	Sensor
Ear-O-Smart	Ear	Pulse oximeter
Cosinuss	Ear	Pulse oximeter
Earphone	Ear	Pulse oximeter (Bragi)
Watch	Hand/Wrist	Pulse oximeter (e.g., Samsung Gear Fit, Basis)
Fingertip	Fingertip	Pulse oximeter (e.g., Go2 Fingertip Pulse Oximeter
Sensor patch	Hand	Electrocardiogram (Avery Dennison Metria)
Wristband	Wrist	Touch-activated electrocardiogram sensor (e.g., Phyode W/Me wristband)
Wristband		Pressure Sensor (e.g., iHealth, Omron)
Glass	Head	Gyroscope, accelerometer, image sensor (e.g., Google Glass)
Shirt	Torso	3D accelerometer (e.g., PoloTech)

3.2.2 Respiration Rate

Monitoring of respiration rate is one of the fundamental parameters for governing the patient's well-being during medical checkup (AL-Khalidi et al., 2011). Continuous monitoring of respiration rate can help the clinicians predict the progression of several critical illnesses, such as cardiac arrest and lung diseases like chronic obstructive pulmonary disease (COPD) (Vashist et al., 2014), which is one of the major ailments in geriatric population affecting almost 210 million people across the globe (WHO, 2007).

The examination of this parameter in athletics also assists in attaining better respiratory performance (Elliott and Coventry, 2012; Chan et al., 2012; Teng et al., 2008). Majorly, the respiration rate is assessed via two modes: (a) contact mode (Sharma et al., 2015; Addison et al., 2015), through patching the sensing devices to the body and (b) noncontact mode (32 AR), using infrared-based sensors to capture images of the patients. Some examples of wearable devices in the form of patches, shirts, and bracelets for monitoring of respiration rate are given in Table 3.2. Additionally, various sensor-based devices have been developed to monitor the medical condition of COPD patients (Belza et al., 2001; Moy et al., 2003; Sherrill et al., 2005; Steele et al., 2000; Atallah et al., 2010; Koul et al., 2013). These advancements in the wearable devices enabled the patients to continuously monitor their condition at home, thus minimizing the risk of other hospital-acquired infections.

The three methods that are widely used for this analysis are (i) elastomeric plethysmography (EP), which generally uses an elastic belt to convert the current

TABLE 3.2
Overview of Commercially Available Wearable Devices for Measurement of Respiration Rate (Koydemir and Ozcan, 2018)

Wearable device	Body parts	Sensor
Belt accessory (e.g., Spire)	Torso	Accelerometer
Smart textile electrocardiogram sensor	Torso	Piezo-resistive sensor
Glass	Head	Accelerometer, image sensor, gyroscope

variation of piezoelectric sensors into voltage, (ii) impedance plethysmography (IP), which uses impedance changes of the body surface caused by expansion and contraction during breathing, and (iii) respiratory inductive plethysmography (RIP) principle, which is based on a loop wire with current that produces magnetic field normal to the loop orientation. Besides these methods, other alternative technologies like pulse oximetry, optical fibers, accelerometers, polymer-based transducers, etc. are used to determine the respiratory waveform (AL-Khalidi et al., 2011, Emmanouilidou et al., 2012).

3.2.3 Body Temperature

Body temperature measurement is another significant parameter or sign of interest incorporated in the wearable devices as an increase in body temperature is crucial indicator for any possible infections or disturbances in the immunological system of users. It is always preferable to measure body (core) temperature rather than the skin temperature as it gets affected by many external parameters like ambient temperature, humidity, etc (WHO, 2015). Since the fluctuation in body temperature is very low, therefore it is measured in not-so-frequent certain time intervals (Koydemir and Ozcan, 2018).

Table 3.3 lists the numerous wearable systems available in the market to measure body temperatures (Popovic et al., 2014; Webb et al., 2013). For example, the device ECTemp has been developed to measure real-time core temperature with

TABLE 3.3
Overview of Some Commercially Available Wearable Devices for Measurement of Body Temperature (Koydemir and Ozcan, 2018)

Wearable device	Body parts	Sensor
Earpiece (e.g., Cosinuss one earpiece)	Head	Temperature
Tattoo (e.g., VivaLnk Fever Scout)	Torso	Temperature
Earphone (Bragi)	Head	Temperature
Watch (e.g., Basi)	Wrist	Temperature

high accuracy rate and has tremendous application in military defense field (Looney et al., 2018).

3.2.4 Blood Pressure

Blood pressure is one of the vital cardiopulmonary parameters where the optimum range is 120/80 mm Hg, whereas a value above +10 higher than the normal range indicates that the patient has prehypertension or high blood pressure levels that might damage the walls of the arteries. Therefore, monitoring blood pressure levels at frequent intervals could be useful in preventing and controlling many health complications caused due to high blood pressure, which is reported to play a major role in the global burden of diseases.

The conventional inflatable pressure cuffs with a stethoscope have been reported to cause discomfort, sleep disruption, as well as skin irritations (Leng et al., 2015). To overcome these aforementioned challenges, noninvasive monitoring devices in the form of wrist and arm-based monitors are now available (Table 3.4), which also rule out human errors caused due to the movement of patients while measuring the blood pressure.

3.2.5 Blood Glucose

Measurement of blood glucose level is important for patients suffering from diabetes mellitus, a disease whereby sufficient insulin is not produced by the body (Koydemir and Ozcan, 2018). Diabetes also leads to several physiological clinical manifestations such as cerebral vascular disturbance, retinopathy, and nephropathy. Therefore, clinicians recommend that diabetic individuals need to control the optimum glucose concentration in the body by continuous measuring of glucose levels and injecting insulin whenever needed. A lot of efforts have been taken to avoid the conventional routine pricking method and as a result several wearable noninvasive techniques have been developed that are already commercialized. For instance, methods like bioimpedance spectroscopy for continuous blood glucose monitoring; however, the drawback of this nonviable technique is its poor reliability and acquisition requirements (So et al., 2012).

TABLE 3.4
Important Commercially Available Wearable Devices for Measurement of Blood Pressure (Koydemir and Ozcan, 2018)

Wearable device	Body parts	Sensor
Sensor	Torso	Two photoplethysmography sensors
Patch	Arm	Potential difference
Wristband (e.g., iHealth, Omron)	Arm	Pressure sensor

Similarly, the drawback of another method called electromagnetic sensing is that it is largely affected by the temperature (So et al., 2012). Likewise, fluorescence technology and infrared spectroscopy are both potential technologies but also have inherent shortcomings, namely low penetration and reading correlation, respectively (Takahashi et al., 2013).

A wearable artificial pancreas with a smartphone-enabled application, Genesis (Pancreum, 2015), comprises a flexible core system as a brain and three wedges each for insulin administration, glucose detecting, and glucagon delivery. A new wearable, a smart contact lens, is being developed by Google/Verily Life Sciences in partnership with Novartis to measure blood sugar levels (Elenko et al., 2015).

3.2.6 Blood Oxygen Saturation

The measurement of blood oxygen levels in the vessels is called blood oxygen saturation test and the standard range for the arterial oxygen level is 75–100 mm Hg. Measurement of blood oxygen saturation level is based upon the photoplethysmography (PPG) technology and pulse oximetry principles. The PPG acquires the blood vessel variation waveform to estimate blood oxygen saturation. This is based upon the fact that the hemoglobin absorbance spectrum changes when it binds with oxygen. Similarly, integrating pulse oximeter into wearable devices with light-emitting diodes (LEDs) at two wavelength scans also be employed to measure the blood oxygen saturation level. Generally, two different wavelengths, one less than 810 nm and the other is higher than 810 nm are used in this case. The device is composed of a photodiode which generally lies on the opposite side of the tissue and emits light. The emitted light transmits through the finger or ear and determines the blood oxygen saturation level through a ratio metric analysis of the oxygen and deoxygenated blood hemoglobin in reference to a pre-determined calibration curve. However, accurate measurement of blood oxygen saturation in anemic patients is still a big challenge (Koydemir and Ozcan, 2018; Dias and Paulo Silva, 2018).

3.2.7 Motion Evaluation

Determination of body movements and motions has wide applications in healthcare and sports domain. The most popular wearable wristband-style commercial motion trackers are mentioned in Table 3.5 (Haghi et al., 2017). These smartphone-enabled devices may provide real-time digital activity measurement information (Anliker et al., 2004). Also, they enable the wearer to calculate the distance walked, which is very useful to ensure that the user maintains sufficient physical activity every day to lead a healthy life.

The principle of motion tracking is also useful in physiotherapy to evaluate specific therapeutic exercise movements, thereby maximizing patient's recovery (Anliker et al., 2004). In particular, three-axis accelerometers, magnetometers, and gyroscopes sensors are used to accurately observe motion and human activity recognition and the combination of these three sensors leads to 9 DoF. Due to the high risk of falls reported in geriatric population, motion-sensing trackers are also nowadays largely used for fall detection.

TABLE 3.5
Comparative Analysis of Features of Four Common Commercial Wearable Devices (Haghi et al., 2017)

Device	Communication mode	Price ($)	Weight (g)	Battery life (month)	Rechargeable battery	Dimension
Fitbit Flex	Wireless-connection to mobile application only	100	16.4	4–6	Yes	6.3 × 8.2
Withings Pulse	Wi-Fi-enabled	120	8	6	Yes	1.7 × 0.87 × 0.33
Misfit Shine	Compatible with Android as well as the iPhone	100	9.4	3	No	1.08 × 0.13 × 1.08
Jawbone	Bluetooth	100	19	4–6	Yes	6.1 × 6.1

3.2.8 Other Biomedical Applications of Wearable Devices

- DentiTrac (Braebon, 2015; Bradley, 2015) is an FDA-approved oral device used to monitor sleep apnea, which is extremely common among people.
- The Vega GPS bracelet is a wearable GPS in-built device for mobile communications positioning and monitoring the location of patients having a medical condition called dementia such as Alzheimer's disease, Parkinson's disease, and also epilepsy (Everon, 2015). For example, Embrace by Empatica (Milan, Italy) is used for monitoring the vital physiological signals in epileptic people (Koydemir and Ozcan, 2018).
- Kite Patch is a patch-based wearable device which can disperse volatile compounds and can be worn on dress to repel mosquitoes (KitePatch, 2018; Turner et al., 2011).
- Wearable wristband UV sensors can be used to monitor UV exposure levels along with assessing vitamin D concentration in the body.
- A wearable smart glass coined Eyes-On technology (Evena Med, 2015), which employs multispectral 3D imaging and uses infrared sensors, enables clinicians to rapidly locate patients' veins. Likewise, Alpha-Fit GmbH (Wertheim, Germany) developed Smart socks which can provide data related to the 3D dynamic pressure distribution over the foot area while the user is walking. This data plays a significant role in designing customized shoes for patients with diabetic foot syndrome (Munro et al., 2008; Alphafit, 2015; Esfahani and Nussbaum, 2018).
- The researchers and scientists at University of Michigan developed a wearable device which is capable of collecting and examining tumor cells in the blood continuously (Kim et al., 2019). This wrist-worn device can screen patients'

blood for a certain duration of time to procure the circulating tumor cells of interest (Hyun et al., 2019). This innovative device offers a promising approach for convenient detection of cancers without deploying extensive invasive procedures like tissue biopsy (Brannon-Peppas and Blanchette, 2014).

- The human sweat is an important body fluid which can be used to retrieve various physiological conditions of the human body in a noninvasive approach. Over the years a lot of efforts have been made to develop a noninvasive approach to detect the sweat analyte concentration (Gao et al., 2016). Center for Bio-Integrated Electronics at Northwestern University, Chicago developed a sweat sensor which can monitor the physiological condition of the human body by detecting different analytes like – lactate, glucose, chloride, and pH (Peppas et al. 2000). Furthermore, the sensor has the potential to measure the sweat rate and sweat loss as well (Wilson, 2019).
- Peritoneal dialysis and hemodialysis are the most common practices for the treatment of renal failure. These procedures are inconvenient for the patients and requires professional interventions. To overcome this problem, AWAK Technologies developed a wearable and portable peritoneal dialysis device coined as AWAK PD, which can perform dialysis on the go reducing the dependency on inconvenient therapies and treatments (Doc wire news, 2019).

3.3 FEW EXAMPLES OF INNOVATIVE WEARABLE HEALTHCARE DEVICES CURRENTLY UNDER DEVELOPMENT

3.3.1 RespiroGear – Respiratory Rate Controller

3.3.1.1 Background

COPDs account for 20% of the total mortality rate in India. Increasing air pollution across the country contributes significantly to the rising number of COPD patients. Death due to COPD is because of lack of improper dose of medication or inhaler during an asthma attack. Innovative solutions like a clip-on device where the doses/sprays of inhaler would be set automatically according to the reading of spirometer. Also, if a person is under a sudden, severe asthmatic attack and in case there are no doctors to consult about the doses of inhaler, then this device would automatically determine the inhaler dose and help save the patient's life. In the recent years, several efforts have been made to develop devices which can deliver pharmaceutical preparations to the oral cavity. Earlier the solution was to use a propellant to discharge powdered medication into the oral cavity of the patient. The extensive usage of a propellant could be harmful to the environment and aggravate a patient's pre-existing bronchial condition. To overcome this situation, Pritam Dhalla (co-author of this chapter) and his team are developing an inhalation-based device named as RespiroGear (Figure 3.3) at KIIT - Technology Business Incubator, (KIIT-TBI), Bhubaneswar, India.

3.3.1.2 Novelty

This combined automatic device would reduce the dependency of patients on doctors during chronic COPD or specially in an emergency and save a large number of patient's lives. The present invention relates generally to an inhaler, and more

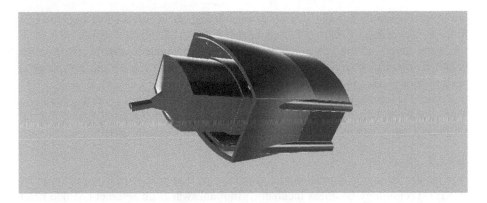
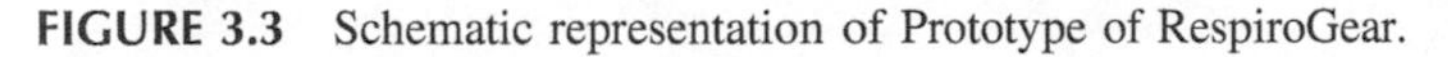

FIGURE 3.3 Schematic representation of Prototype of RespiroGear.

specifically to an inhaler with mouthpiece adapter and a patient feedback mechanism. The mouthpiece adapter and patient feedback mechanism of the present invention is used in an inhaler such as a dry powder inhaler DPI to facilitate use of the inhaler in pediatric, elderly, and susceptible patients. The present invention can be used in other applications such as a Metered Dose Inhaler (MDI).

3.3.1.3 Core Technology

This technology introduces a clip-on smart inhaler that enables any ordinary inhaler to function with more efficiency. With a rapid spike in the number of patients diagnosed with pulmonary diseases, the scope of this device is huge as the efficiency of all other available products is reasonably less. Whether an MDI can deliver the correct amount of medication to the lungs depends on the skill of the person using it. That means whether or not the medicine is correctly released depends on whether the MDI user is dexterous, can use the body well in coordination, has the timing, or is skilled. This can be a big complication for young patients because of the issue of not being able to use their body well, especially if there is inflammation in the respiratory tract. For regular treatment of asthma symptoms, MDIs are the most widely prescribed medication delivery system for inhaled medications for asthmatics. For symptomatic relief and proper control of the disease, almost all the asthma patients depend on the usage of MDIs. Despite the regular use of MDIs, a high percentage of users incorrectly employ MDIs. MPV of this product is ready and now the product is under clinical trials.

3.3.2 CardioMate – Heart Rate and Activity Monitoring for Disease Diagnosis

3.3.2.1 Background

Cardiovascular diseases (CVDs) are leading cause of deaths globally. India contributes to 20%–35% of the global mortality rate due to CVDs (Mozaffarian et al., 2015). The figure is worse in rural sector, but does not come into limelight due to under-reporting and incorrect diagnosis. One primary reason for this is that it is not possible or feasible to have costly equipment or trained human resource for preliminary screening of heart problems at the Public Healthcare Centers (PHCs) or subcenter level and there is no technology that can enable ANM/ASHA/frontline health workers to screen people with such problem at the last mile. So, what is needed here is a technology that can be used for screening of heart diseases at the last mile. The technology must be low in cost, fairly easy to use, and interpretation should be easy without requiring complex training such that it can be used in rural settings or by frontline workers directly (Rajala and Lekkala, 2010).

3.3.2.2 Novelty

Against this backdrop another device (Figure 3.4) that is being developed in house at KIIT-Technology Business Incubator, Bhubaneswar is an Internet-enabled heart monitoring device:

- It is as compact as a smartphone and costs around 1/10 of any standard ECG machine.
- It is very easy to use and requires minimal training: All you have to do is place it on the chest, leave it there for a minute and it would deliver the result in the form of a simple message on the screen whether the patient's heart is normal or there is a probability of an underlying heart disease, so that they can be referred for further analysis.
- The entire procedure is voice-guided for ease of the user and thus personnels do not have to go through any complex training.
- This can be used by ASHA or frontline workers or at PHC/Sub center level for preliminary screening of heart disease and refer up patients accordingly.

3.3.2.3 Core Technology

The USP and the core technology is based upon the fact that besides capturing ECG, it also captures heart murmurs and combines both these data points to predict the probability of an underlying heart disease. Innovators are intending to build a product which can be used for screening heart conditions in humans. It would include an ECG module, heart murmur module, and Artificial Intelligence (AI) for crunching this data to predict presence of a certain heart disease. The device would

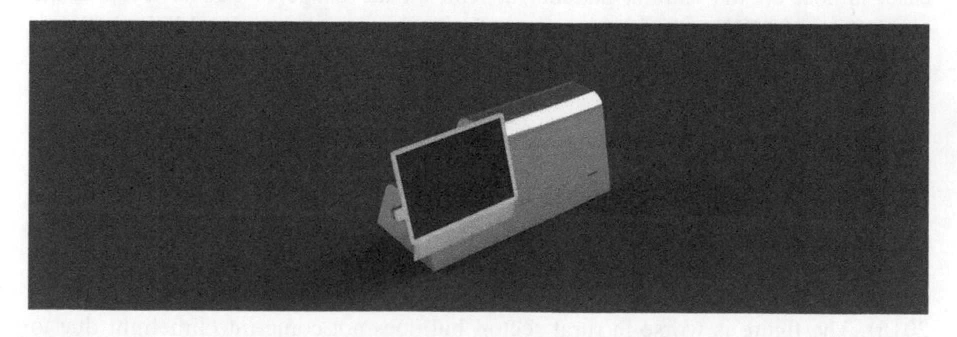

FIGURE 3.4 Schematic representation of Prototype of CardioMate.

be battery operated and would have a touch-enabled display, making it easy to use in the last mile. First phase trial of this product is already done and now the device is ready for market entry and further evaluation from market survey.

3.4 KEY FACTORS INFLUENCING THE GROWTH OF HEALTHCARE DEVICE SECTOR, PARTICULARLY IN THE INDIA CONTEXT

With the recent upsurge in scientific and technology breakthroughs, the pace of medical invention is exponentially increasing, however as the demand rises, supply needs to keep pace. Factors affecting the growth of healthcare device sector are discussed in this section:

a. **Rising Chronic Disease:** In the present-day scenario, India has been burdened with highest number of communicable diseases in the world, however, even today; the majority of India's population cannot afford anything better than the most basic healthcare. Therefore, medical devices are needed to make healthcare both affordable and accessible to a larger percentage of the population (Bagcchi, 2015). This is possible by constant monitoring of health indicators remotely through wearable devices. These wearable devices and mobile apps now have been integrated with telemedicine to structure the medical Internet of Things.
b. **Increased life expectancy and aging population:** Advancements in the medical field have led to a sharp increase in life expectancy causing increase in the proportion of aged population. This is consequently creating upward pressure on the demand for medical care. It is expected that the population above 65 years will increase from 5% in 2005 to 15% by 2030 (https://www.un.org/en/development/desa/population/publications/pdf/ageing/WPA2015_Report.pdf). Hence, many people are seeking for an alternative, such as a device that can be worn on the body, which would not only continuously monitor the user's health in real time but also provide timely insights into various health parameters to the user as well as his or her clinician (Martini and Bartholomew, 2012).
c. **Increasing awareness:** The Indian consumer is becoming more aware today about the recent modern medical technologies and equipment available in the market, and consequently demanding the same (Deloitte, 2017). At the same time, awareness about regular monitoring of health parameters for prevention of any future disease through advertisements, training, and education workshops/seminars, etc. have resulted in increased demand for many wearable devices like fit bands, smart watches, smart fabrics, orthopedic shoes, etc (Markets and Markets, 2016).

3.5 CHALLENGES AND WAY FORWARD OF WEARABLE DEVICES IN HEALTHCARE TECHNOLOGY

Wearable devices in recent years have undergone various developments in terms of low-power integrated circuits, wireless communications, extreme miniaturization, lighter, and have longer battery lives along with good sensitivity and specificity (Yilmaz et al., 2010). Nonetheless, several challenges still need to be addressed for deployment of wearables in market (Bazaka and Jacob, 2013). This sections briefly reviews the current limitations of wireless and sensor-integrated wearable devices and discusses various countermeasures against them.

a. **Security:** The security of the data collection and analysis is a pivotal issue in any wireless sensor, for use in healthcare domain (Kim et al., 2015). Since wearables are small devices which can store large volume of data, therefore, development of more secure and robust integrated systems with access control is needed (Dey et al., 2019).
b. **Sensitivity of sensors:** The sensitivity of the wearables is most vital when users, particularly athletes, use these devices under varying environmental conditions such as humid or warm temperature. Therefore, highly sensitive sensors are required that would allow continuous monitoring of body health parameters while not compromising optimum performance during running, swimming, depending on targeted application. Wearable smart clothes need to be washable and flexible that do not break while stretching or folding (Iqbal et al., 2016).
c. **Low power consumption:** Battery life of sensors is a key hurdle in wearable health devices and deeply seeks investigations and solutions (Lundager et al., 2016; Darwish and Hassanien, 2011). We still need robust solutions like designing battery less scavenging energy from human or environment such as the new "green technology" which harnesses the solar energy through miniature solar cells.
d. **User-friendly:** For the wearables to gain wide utility, both the healthcare professionals as well as the end users should find the device very easy to use. The needs for different category of end users like geriatric population, cognitive disabled, or patients with other disabilities should be kept into considerations while developing the system.
e. **Biocompatibility:** The hardware and electronic components of the device should comply with the biocompatibility aspect for medical and biological applications (Kim et al., 2015). Testing of this bio-stability is often challenging, especially for long-term implants (Koydemir and Ozcan et al., 2018).
f. **Accessibility:** In low- and middle-income countries, a majority of the population resides in the rural areas or remote locations. These areas are deprived of various important factors like modern wireless infrastructure, technical expertise, etc. which could potentially become a stumbling block for efficient performance of the device in the rural settings. Furthermore, the high cost of the wearable devices makes it more challenging in terms of affordability in the rural and urban settings.
g. **Affordability:** One of the major challenges in enabling the wearable devices in the healthcare system is its high initial investment and maintenance cost, which makes it difficult to setup in the rural settings (FICCI, 2016). Implementation of these wearable devices in healthcare technology requires focus on developing low-cost solutions to adopt the solution at a larger scale efficiently.

It is worthwhile to mention that in addition to development of innovative products for healthcare application, the entire pipeline from product development to commercialization needs to be symmetrically strategized in the medical technology ecosystem. Furthermore, for innovation to make an impact, all stakeholders need to strategize and move forward together for actions to resonate and bring about a revolutionary change in the healthcare sector (Inc42, 2018).

REFERENCES

Aarts V, Dellimore KH, Wijshoff R, Derkx R, van de Laar J, Muehlsteff J. Performance of an accelerometer-based pulse presence detection approach compared to a reference sensor. In 2017 IEEE 14th International Conference on Wearable and Implantable Body Sensor Networks (BSN). 2017 May (pp. 165–168). IEEE.

Addison PS, Watson JN, Mestek ML, Ochs JP, Uribe AA, Bergese SD. Pulse oximetry-derived respiratory rate in general care floor patients. *Journal of Clinical Monitoring and Computing*. 2015 Feb 1;29(1):113–120.

AL-Khalidi FQ, Saatchi R, Burke D, Elphick H, Tan S. Respiration rate monitoring methods: A review. *Pediatric Pulmonology*. 2011 Jun;46(6):523–529.

Alphafit. *Smart sock*. 2015. http://www.alpha-fit.de/en/products/smartsock.html

Anliker U, Ward JA, Lukowicz P, Troster G, Dolveck F, Baer M, Keita F, Schenker EB, Catarsi F, Coluccini L, Belardinelli A. AMON: A wearable multiparameter medical monitoring and alert system. *IEEE Transactions on Information Technology in Biomedicine*. 2004 Nov 30;8(4):415–427.

Atallah L, Zhang J, Lo BP, Shrikrishna D, Kelly JL, Jackson A, Polkey MI, Yang GZ, Hopkinson NS. Validation of an ear worn sensor for activity monitoring in COPD. In A27. Advances in Pulmonary Rehabilitation. 2010 May (pp. A1211–A1211). American Thoracic Society.

Bagcchi S. India has low doctor to patient ratio, study finds. *British Medical Journal*. 2015; 351:h5195.

Bazaka K, Jacob MV. Implantable devices: Issues and challenges. *Electronics*. 2013 Mar; 2(1):1–34.

Belza B, Steele BG, Hunziker J, Lakshminaryan S, Holt L, Buchner DM. Correlates of physical activity in chronic obstructive pulmonary disease. *Nursing Research*. 2001 Jul 1;50(4):195–202.

Bhatt C, Dey N, Ashour AS, eds. Internet of things and big data technologies for next generation healthcare. 2017. Springer International Publishing.

Bradley DC, inventor; Braebon Medical Corp, assignee. Method and apparatus for verifying compliance with dental appliance therapy. *United States patent application US 14/111,079*. 2015 Apr 23.

Braebon. DentiTrac. 2015. https://www.braebon.com/products/dentitrac/

Brannon-Peppas L, Blanchette JO. Nanoparticle and targeted systems for cancer therapy. *Advanced Drug Delivery Reviews*. 2004 Sep 22;56(11):1649–1659.

Chan L, Hsieh CH, Chen YL, Yang S, Huang DY, Liang RH, Chen BYCyclops: Wearable and single-piece full-body gesture input devices. In Proceedings of the 33rd Annual ACM Conference on Human Factors in Computing Systems. 2015. (pp. 3001–3009).

Deloitte. Medical technology industry in India: Riding the growth curve. 2010. https://www2.deloitte.com/content/dam/Deloitte/in/Documents/life-sciences-health-care/in-lshc-medical-technology-in-India-noexp.pdf

Deloitte. Medical device industry in India: The evolving landscape, opportunities and challenges. 2017. https://www2.deloitte.com/in/en/pages/life-sciences-and-healthcare/articles/medical-technology-industry-in-india.html

Dey N, Ashour AS, Fong SJ, Bhatt C, eds. *Wearable and implantable medical devices: applications and challenges*. 2019 Sep 6. Academic Press.

Dey N, Ashour AS, Shi F, Fong SJ, Sherratt RS. Developing residential wireless sensor networks for ECG healthcare monitoring. *IEEE Transactions on Consumer Electronics*. 2017 Nov;63(4):442–449.

Dias D, Paulo Silva Cunha J. Wearable health devices—vital sign monitoring, systems and technologies. *Sensors*. 2018 Aug;18(8):2414.

Doc wire news. World's first wearable peritoneal dialysis device receives FDA breakthrough status by Jack Carfagno. 2019. https://www.docwirenews.com/docwire-pick/future-of-medicine-picks/worlds-firstwearable-peritoneal-dialysis-device-receives-fda-breakthrough-status/

Elenko E, Underwood L, Zohar D. Defining digital medicine. *Nature Biotechnology*. 2015 May;33(5):456–461.

Elliott M, Coventry A. Critical care: The eight vital signs of patient monitoring. *British Journal of Nursing*. 2012 May 23;21(10):621–625.

Emmanouilidou D, Patil K, West J, Elhileli M. A multiresolution analysis for detection of abnormal lung sounds. In Conference Proceedings of IEEE Engineering in Medicine and Biology Society. 2012 (pp. 3139–3142). IEEE.

Evena Med. Eyes-on glasses 3.0. 2015. https://evenamed.com/eyes-on-glasses/

Everon. Vega GPS Bracelet. 2015. https://everon.fi/en/solutions/vega-gps-safety-solution-andbracelet

Esfahani MIM, Nussbaum MA, Preferred placement and usability of a smart textile system vs. inertial measurement units for activity monitoring. *Sensors*. 2018; 18(8), 2501.

FICCI. Assessment of factors determining accessibility of medical devices in India 2020. http://ficci.in/spdocument/20211/FICCI-F&S-Report-on-Medical-Devices.pdf

FICCI. Report on Indian healthcare startups: An inside look into funding. 2016. https://assets.kpmg/content/dam/kpmg/in/pdf/2016/09/FICCI-Heal.pdf

Gao W, Emaminejad S, Wu E, Davies ZA, Nyein HYY, Challa S, Davis RW. Autonomous sweat extraction and analysis applied to cystic fibrosis and glucose monitoring using a fully integrated wearable platform. *Proceedings of the national academy of sciences*. 2017;114(18), 4625–4530.

Giovangrandi L, Inan OT, Banerjee D, Kovacs GT. Preliminary results from BCG and ECG measurements in the heart failure clinic. In 2012 Annual International Conference of the IEEE Engineering in Medicine and Biology Society. 2012 Aug 28 (pp. 3780–3783). IEEE.

Haghi M, Thurow K, Stoll R. Wearable devices in medical internet of things: Scientific research and commercially available devices. *Healthcare Informatics Research*. 2017 Jan 1;23(1):4–15.

Haghi M, Thurow K, Stoll N. A multi-tasking, multi-layer and replaceable wrist-worn environmental monitoring sensor node. In 5th International Conference on Control, Decision and Information Technologies (CoDIT). 2018. (pp. 25–31).

Hayward J, Chansin G, Zervos H. Wearable technology 2017–2027: Markets, players, forecasts. *IDTexEx Report*. 2017.

Inc42. Indian tech startup funding report. 2018. https://pages.inc42.com/wp-content/uploads/woocommerce_uploads/2018/01/Inc42-Annual-Funding-Report-2018.pdf

Iqbal MH, Aydin A, Brunckhorst O, Dasgupta P, Ahmed K. A review of wearable technology in medicine. *Journal of the Royal Society of Medicine*. 2016 Oct;109(10): 372–380.

Joshi M, Ashrafian H, Aufegger L, Khan S, Arora S, Cooke G, Darzi A. Wearable sensors to improve detection of patient deterioration. *Expert Review of Medical Devices*. 2019 Feb 1;16(2):145–154.

Kim TH, Wang Y, Oliver CR, Thamm DH, Cooling L, Paoletti C, Smith KJ, Nagrath S, Hayes DF. A temporary indwelling intravascular aphaeretic system for in vivo enrichment of circulating tumor cells. *Nature Communications*. 2019 Apr 1;10(1):1–8.

Kim Y, Lee W, Raghunathan A, Raghunathan V, Jha NK. Reliability and security of implantable and wearable medical devices. *In implantable biomedical microsystems*. 2015 Jan 1 (pp. 167–199). William Andrew Publishing.

KitePatch. *Kite patch*. 2018. http://www.kitepatch.com/kite-patch/

Koul PA. Chronic obstructive pulmonary disease: Indian guidelines and the road ahead. *Lung India*. 2013;175–177.

Koydemir HC, Ozcan A. Wearable and implantable sensors for biomedical applications. *Annual Review of Analytical Chemistry*. 2018 Jun 12;11:127–146.

Leng S, Tan RS, Chai KTC, Wang C, Ghista D, Zhong L. The electronic stethoscope. *BioMedical Engineering OnLine*. 2015;14:66.

Looney DP, Buller MJ, Gribok AV, Leger JL, Potter AW, Rumpler WV, Tharion WJ, Welles AP, Friedl KE, Hoyt RW. Estimating resting core temperature using heart rate. Journal for the Measurement of Physical *Behaviour*. 2018 Jun 1;1(2):79–86.

Lundager K, Zeinali B, Tohidi M, Madsen JK, Moradi F. Low power design for future wearable and implantable devices. *Journal of Low Power Electronics and Applications*. 2016 Dec;6(4):20.

Markets and Markets. Point-of-care diagnostic market worth $27.5 billion by 2018. 2016. http://www.marketsandmarkets.com/PressReleases/point-of-care-diagnostic.asp.

Martini F, Bartholomew EF. *Studyguide for essentials of anatomy and physiology*. 2012. Academic Internet Publishers.

Moy ML, Mentzer SJ, Reilly JJ. Ambulatory monitoring of cumulative free-living activity. *IEEE Engineering in Medicine and Biology Magazine*. 2003 Jul 22;22(3):89–95.

Mozaffarian D, Benjamin EJ, Go AS, Arnett DK, Blaha MJ, et al. Heart disease and stroke statistics—2015 update. Circulation. 2015;131(4).

Munro BJ, Campbell TE, Wallace GG, Steele JR. The intelligent knee sleeve: A wearable biofeedback device. *Sensors and Actuators B: Chemical*. 2008 May 14;131(2):541–547.

Nair AG, Kamal S, Dave TV, Mishra K, Reddy HS, Della Rocca D, Della Rocca RC, Andron A, Jain V. Surgeon point-of-view recording: Using a high-definition head-mounted video camera in the operating room. *Indian Journal of Ophthalmology*. 2015 Oct;63(10):771.

Olmez T, Dokur Z. Classification of heart sounds using an artificial neural network. *Pattern Recognition Letters*. 2003:617–629.

Ozcan A. Mobile phones democratize and cultivate next-generation imaging, diagnostics and measurement tools. *Lab on a Chip*. 2014;14(17):3187–3194.

Pancreum. *Wearable pancreas*. 2015. http://pancreum.com/index.html

Peppas NA, Huang Y, Torres-Lugo M, Ward JH, Zhang J. Physicochemical foundations and structural design of hydrogels in medicine and biology. *Annual Review of Biomedical Engineering*. 2000 Aug;2(1):9–29.

Popovic Z, Momenroodaki P, Scheeler R. Toward wearable wireless thermometers for internal body temperature measurements. *IEEE Communications Magazine*. 2014 Oct 9;52(10):118–125.

Rajala S, Lekkala J. Film-type sensor materials PVDF and EMFi in measurement of cardiorespiratory signals—A review. *IEEE Sensors Journal*. 2010:439–446.

Sharma H, Sharma KK, Bhagat OL. Respiratory rate extraction from single-lead ECG using homomorphic filtering. *Computers in Biology and Medicine*. 2015 Apr 1;59:80–86.

Sherrill DM, Moy ML, Reilly JJ, Bonato P. Using hierarchical clustering methods to classify motor activities of COPD patients from wearable sensor data. *Journal of NeuroEngineering and Rehabilitation*. 2005 Dec;2(1):16.

So CF, Choi KS, Wong TK, Chung JW. Recent advances in noninvasive glucose monitoring. *Medical Devices (Auckland, NZ)*. 2012;5:45.

Stahl SE, An HS, Dinkel DM, Noble JM, Lee JM. How accurate are the wrist-based heart rate monitors during walking and running activities? Are they accurate enough? *BMJ Open Sport & Exercise Medicine*. 2016 Apr 1;2(1):e000106.

Steele BG, Holt L, Belza B, Ferris S, Lakshminaryan S, Buchner DM. Quantitating physical activity in COPD using a triaxial accelerometer. *Chest.* 2000 May 1;117(5):1359–1367.

Takahashi M, Heo YJ, Kawanishi T, Okitsu T, Takeuchi S. Portable continuous glucose monitoring systems with implantable fluorescent hydrogel microfibers. In 2013 IEEE 26th International Conference on Micro Electro Mechanical Systems (MEMS). 2013 Jan 20 (pp. 1089–1092). IEEE.

Teng XF, Zhang YT, Poon CC, Bonato P. Wearable medical systems for p-health. *IEEE Reviews in Biomedical Engineering*. 2008 Dec 12;1:62–74.

Turner SL, Li N, Guda T, Githure J, Cardé RT, Ray A. Ultra-prolonged activation of CO2-sensing neurons disorients mosquitoes. *Nature.* 2011 Jun;474(7349):87–91.

Vashist SK, Mudanyali O, Schneider EM, Zengerle R, Ozcan A. Cellphone-based devices for bioanalytical sciences. *Analytical and Bioanalytical Chemistry*. 2014 May 1;406(14): 3263–3277.

Webb RC, Bonifas AP, Behnaz A, Zhang Y, Yu KJ, Cheng H, Shi M, Bian Z, Liu Z, Kim YS, Yeo WH. Ultrathin conformal devices for precise and continuous thermal characterization of human skin. *Nature Materials*. 2013 Oct;12(10):938–944.

WHO. *Global surveillance, prevention and control of chronic respiratory diseases: a comprehensive approach* 2007. WHO.

WHO. Skin cancers. 2015. WHO. www.who.int/uv/faq/skincancer/en/index1.html

Wilson EK. Wearable sweat sensors. *Engineering*. 2019 Jul 11;5(3):359–360.

Yilmaz T, Foster R, Hao Y. Detecting vital signs with wearable wireless sensors. *Sensors.* 2010 Dec;10(12):10837–10862.

Zhang W, Guo X, Yuan H, Zhu X. Heart sound classification and recognition based on EEMD and correlation dimension. *Journal of Mechanics in Medicine and Biology. 2014*;14(4):1450046.

4 Advancements in Digital Computation: Issues and Opportunities in Healthcare Services

Mayur Rathi[1], S. P. Sonavane[1], S. G. Tamhankar[2], and F. S. Kazi[3]
[1]IT Department, Walchand College of Engineering, Sangli (MS), India
[2]Electronics Department, Walchand College of Engineering, Sangli (MS), India
[3]Electrical Department, V. J. T. I Matunga, Mumbai, India

CONTENTS

4.1 INTRODUCTION

The proposed model is designed to enhance the efficiency of healthcare system against pandemic diseases. The biosensor-based architecture is proposed to collect, process, and sample the data values. The multivalued real-time attributes are heart rate, respiration rate, and temperature to monitor using edge devices with least distance. The Bluetooth network is indeed a transmission network used in an edge device. The multi-parametric attributes are exclusively synchronized with threshold. In today's era, GPS-enabled mobile devices are commonly carried at every location. The activity and spatial information of any patient is a greedy need in pandemic diseases to avoid the outbreak. The real-time data are fetched from biosensors with

DOI: 10.1201/9781003198796-4

cloud-based architecture to adhere the data processing and reliable access over the remote locations [1]. Data polling with mobile devices generates various forms of the data for different time duration to generalize the user profile in day-to-day life. The edge computing functionality can rapidly process data at the intermediate gateway of transmission at the patient side.

The communication medium is optimized with edge computing to preprocess the data at client side. The edge device is a load balancer for medical database systems on the cloud. The sensor patch is synchronized and customized with mobile devices to carry the information with two-way communication [2].

In general, the study of various healthcare systems concentrates mainly on the computing model that handles data with respect to the application. The performance of the system solely depends on the computing model to enhance the outcome in the required form. The medical cloud-based system provides fast, reliable, and accessible multi-tenant service to the clients. Data processing substantially provides dialogues in the healthcare system to signify the treatment of patients with specific guidelines. The availability of symptomatic information allows medical practitioners to treat the patient for cure. The multi-parametric attributes tend to classify the preliminary severity index of the patient. The prominent approach towards the remote access reduces the breakdown rate to maiden stage and prevents the competence of the infection.

The learning model in the training phase is exercised with edge data to sample the data in the classifier. The normal distributions of classes are determined with standard deviation of sampled values for a given interval of time. The confidence curve is the determinant of severity of the patient after monitoring the stream of inputs at cloud. The majority of the samples are unambiguously determined with recommendation to pandemic test. The algorithmic approach is proposed to determine the panic state for outbreak in spreading of the disease. The real-time data model is integrated with behavioral and medical information of users to improve the performance of the system. The finite check of sequence is performed in a medical database system to correlate the client's earlier data with current data. The standard outcome of the classifier can predict the testing with precautionary recommendation for instance data. A case study is discussed to address the contemporary application of the proposed model. The limitations of current healthcare systems are discussed with solution space for differentiated instances of time [2].

The motivation behind this chapter is to provide a remote platform to decide the early measures with classification of patients. The classification adheres the samples into sub-categories of severity index with polling of data from biosensor. The objective behind the study is to provide the pattern-learning platform for pandemic infectious diseases. The normal sequencing and breakdown pattern can be analyzed using a cloud-based data management system. The study emphasized a cost-effective model for testing with severity index of the infection in symptomatic data value from biosensor.

4.2 LITERATURE SURVEY

To propose a model-based system, similar healthcare systems are studied in various domains. The Internet of Things (IOT), Machine Learning (ML), Cloud Computing, and Deep Learning (DL) are the leading technologies to trigger the healthcare system in a real-time environment. The precise outcomes of inter-domain methodologies are discussed with findings and contributions. The common expectation of digital healthcare systems is data processing and prediction models for a random instance.

Several algorithms are studied in regard to propose the computational model in healthcare communication systems. The data models and allied technologies are crucially studied with data preprocessing techniques for various platforms in domains like IOT, blockchain, ML, and cloud systems. The efficiency of network management is studied with prominent effect on client server application to reduce the end-to-end transaction between the user and cloud-based server (Table 4.1).

The alert system is constructed with multivalued data with health sensors in the domain of Internet of Health Sensor Things. The cloud storage improves the processing platform causing least end-to-end delay. The ubiquitous health management system communicates the panic stage of patient to doctors and guardian with data processing exclusively [3]. The virtual platform is proposed

TABLE 4.1
IOT-Based Healthcare Systems with Supporting Techniques

Sr. no	Author	Healthcare system	Methods	Findings and contributions
1	[3]	Big data analytics of IoT-based healthcare monitoring system	IOT and big data analytics	"Internet of health sensor things" is proposed with huge volume of differentiated data handled with HADOOP framework to reduce the response time between end user
2	[4]	A smart platform for personalized healthcare monitoring using semantic technologies	IOT platform integrated with private cloud	It is the heterogeneous system with personalized healthcare with intensive data processing from sources
3	[5]	Smart healthcare system with edge device	IOT-based virtual platform using cloud	Model automates patient data collection, processing, and storage on container with edge device
4	[6]	Empowering healthcare IoT systems with hierarchical edge-based deep learning	Cloud-based IoT system	Demonstrates a real-time health monitoring on ECG classifications
5	[7]	E-Healthcare as a web service	Distributed system with client service architecture	Distributed data management that improves e-healthcare system
6	[8]	Challenges and potential solutions using IoT and big data analytics	IOT and big data analytics	The deployment model for digital healthcare system is proposed with challenges and potential

to collect patient data and process it on the cloud. The edge device is integrated with a container to store and analyze the health record. The IOT-based deep learning edge computing is endorsed in correlation with cloud computing. The patient is monitored continuously as a preventive measure to avoid risk for heart patients [4].

The heterogeneous system collects data from sources to process at private cloud with analytical tools. The real-time health conditions are monitored by doctors and caregivers with an integrated decision-making system. The application is co-ordinated with IOT-based edge devices, SAAS service model, and data analytics [5]. The deployment model for the healthcare system is compared with other models. The comparative model shows that integrated combination of IOT and big data relatively gives more outcome than singular IOT [6,7]. The data analytics for real-time information improves the performance of the decision-making in IOT application [8] (Table 4.2).

TABLE 4.2
Blockchain-Based Healthcare Systems with Supporting Techniques

Sr. no	Author	Healthcare system	Methods	Findings and contributions
1	[9]	A Case Study for Blockchain in Healthcare: Prototype for electronic health records and medical research data	Blockchain and cloud	The blockchain operation that places patient data centrally to preserve the privacy
2	[10]	Blockchain-Based Healthcare Systems	Ethereum-based blockchain	The system highlights the secure and efficient data accessibility in blockchain-based system
3	[11]	Implementing Blockchains for Efficient Health Care: Systematic Review	Blockchain with distributed computing	The model allows a systematic accessibility of data with blockchain as a method of managing healthcare records
4	[12]	MeDShare: Trust-less Medical Data Sharing Among Cloud Service Providers via Blockchain	Blockchain-based cloud healthcare system	The blockchain-based system provides data provenance, auditing, and control for shared medical data in cloud repositories among big data entities
5	[13]	Lightweight Blockchain for Healthcare	Cluster-based blockchain techniques	Faster ledger-based techniques reduce the cost of computation with least transaction time
6	[14]	Blockchain in Healthcare and Health Sciences—A Scoping Review	Blockchain and data analytics	Blockchain impacts electronic data record and privacy in healthcare system

Here are the limitations of IOT-based healthcare systems:

- The centralized system may undermine the security of data.
- Interlopers may get unauthorized access to the system that may laden privacy of the patient.
- The coordination between edge devices may lead to synchronization problems in the system.
- The end-to-end delay between source and destination within application may get affected with IOT edge computing.
- Sensor, network, and device-processing delay may get overwhelmed by the scale data collection from various sources.
- The accuracy of sensors may vary with motion, body temperature, environmental condition that may reduce the accuracy of the system.

Electronic Health Records (EHRs) of patients are surveyed from various locations to perform computation. The decentralized approach assures privacy and security pledge with blockchain mechanism [9]. The primary objective is to secure the data from the public domain to avoid mishandling. The indisputable and easy access to health records are given to the patient exclusively with confidentiality and accountability [10].

The blockchain system is experimented to know the secure ethereum-based transactions to access the data. The ledger technology improves the distributed data management with multi-stakeholder operations [11]. The provisioning of secure channels to transact electronic record between the stakeholders in distributed fashion may overcome the criticism of single point of failure and improves the scalable accessibility [12]. It is the light weight procedure to speed-up the transaction and reduce ledger-updating time for EHR. Patient information is carried in transaction with low-fault tolerance, secured, and high performance ledger to reduce the energy consumption in network transaction [13].

The decentralized ledger approach is proposed with patient involvement in data uploading and access. The decentralized nodes are configured to improve the privacy and timely availability of health records to doctors in an emergency. The tamper-proof system is proposed to design a smart contract in data access mechanism to minimize the risk of data privacy. Data source and auditing methods are discussed with cloud service providers for transition and sharing of information [14] (Table 4.3).

Here are the limitations of blockchain-based healthcare systems:

- Blockchain-based system is not solely sufficient to develop product in healthcare.
- The patient identity has to be revealed at the end in the healthcare systems. That may violate the principle of blockchain technology.
- The locus of healthcare system is treatment of patient with precise accuracy than privacy of health record.
- The data transition and processing is costly and may increase the price of the product.
- The decentralized system requires a node computation and may cause delay in the outcome.

TABLE 4.3
AI&ML-Based Healthcare Systems with Supporting Techniques

Sr. no	Author	Healthcare system	Methods	Findings and contributions
1	[15]	Machine Learning for Improved Diagnosis and Prognosis in Healthcare	Machine learning, image processing, data analytics	Bayesian inference, a paradigm of machine learning, for diagnosing Alzheimer's disease based on cognitive test
2	[16]	Medic: An Artificially Intelligent System to Provide Healthcare Services to Society and Medical Assistance to Doctors	Natural language processing, fuzzy system and deep learning	The application evaluates the health condition to diagnose the patient with deep learning algorithm
3	[18]	A Machine Learning-Based Medical Data Analytics and Visualization Research Platform	Machine learning and data analytics	The machine learning techniques with scale data set are validated in the research. The predictive and prescriptive approach benefited the patient and doctors to provide health measures in precise manner with time being approach
4	[19]	Prediction of Diabetes Using Machine Learning Algorithms in Healthcare	Machine learning with predictive analysis	The comparative study for multiple algorithm for same data set improves the predictive analytics with least computation time
5	[20]	Artificial Intelligence in Healthcare to Train the Patient Before Surgery	Artificial intelligence and machine learning	The conceptual model of artificial intelligence to assist the doctor in training patient before surgery
6	[21]	Cognitive Smart Healthcare for Pathology Detection and Monitoring	Smart sensor network with deep learning	Proposed a decision making system to monitor the state of patient and provide pathology assistance

- The computational power is large. Hence, increases the cost of the transaction.
- The ledger-updating time is large results into low speed-up.

The AI-based assistance is proposed to share a common platform for the doctor and patients. The system manages the patient's appointment, his data training, monitoring before surgery and after surgery [15]. Post-surgery remote access provides the solution by analyzing the health records with blockchain-based data transmission. The IOT-based deep learning is endorsed in correlation with cloud computing [16]. The patient is monitored continuously with measurable body parameters as a preventive measure to avoid any risks. The complete prototype is discussed to diagnose the patient, generation of medical prescription, and recommendation of assistance with the doctor [17]. The delay in treatment is reduced by personalized medical problem-solving algorithms with deep learning-based approaches in the system. The multiple services are provided to doctors for primary inputs to recommend the treatment in emergency situations [18].

The comparative study of a few ML algorithms is discussed with experimental setup on the same predictive data model. The performance and accuracy are discussed for each algorithm with limitations [19].

The multisource data with genomic, behavioral, and clinical sources is processed with ML algorithms to improve the predictive analysis before treatment [20]. The data set includes hereditary characteristics, age, medical history, demographic factor, etc. This improves the automation in healthcare with accuracy towards the predictive model. The neural network is designed to classify the cells to detect breast cancer. The automation is also validated in analysis with real-time multi-attributed data set [21].

Here are the limitations of AI&ML-based healthcare systems:

- The fragmented data may hamper the accuracy of the system.
- State of health data and peripheral inputs are to be cleared before application of AI algorithm.
- The sustainable data access is required to train the system that is lacking in clinical infrastructure.
- ML demands frequent changes in data attributes; may be difficult to provide in health data set.
- Prediction model of AI ML-based system may not be applicable for all categories of users.

4.3 PROPOSED MODEL

The proposed model is consisting of a perception layer, communication layer, and computation layer. Perception layer is measured to sense the data from patients with multiple-valued parameters. The communication layer comprises edge devices to preprocess the data. The computation on structured data is performed to classify the patients in various categories depending on behavioral, medical, and structured data (Figure 4.1).

4.3.1 Overview of the Framework

- **Sensor:** The biosensor to measure the parametric value for symptomatic disease
- **Edge Device:** The mobile device connected with Bluetooth network to sensor with apache flink to process the data
- **Data Storage:** The ultimate storage on medical cloud to store the patient information through android app of the mobile device

4.3.2 Perception Layer

The biosensor patch is fixed on the body of the patient to sense the temperature, heart rate with its variability, and respiratory rate. The behavioral data is streamed

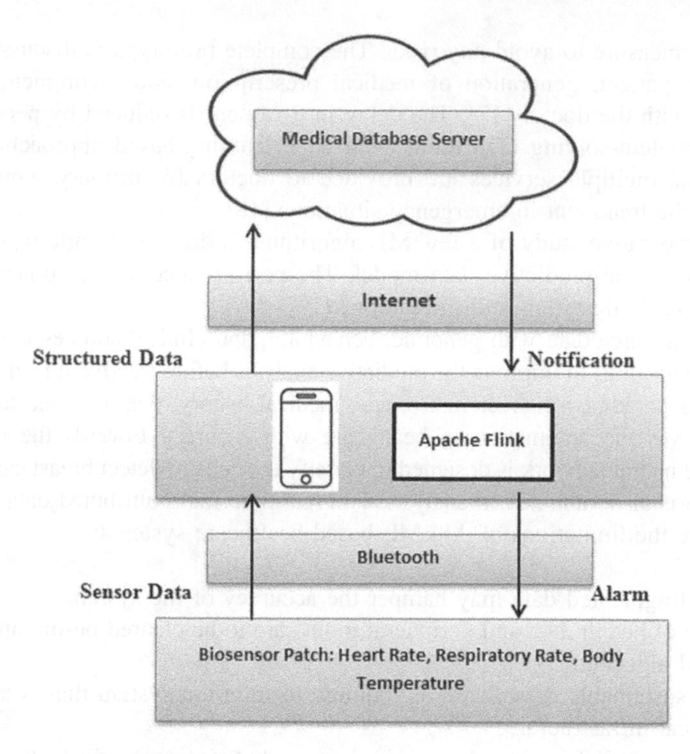

FIGURE 4.1 Biosensor System Overview.

with GPS in mobile devices to record the activity of the patient with latitude and longitude. The medical profile of a patient is mandatorily filled up to generate the medical data. The heart rate is polled for every 3 seconds to monitor the cough. The fluctuations in heart rate are the symptoms of cough and can be verified with respiratory rate. The single biosensor patch consisted of respiratory, temperature, and heart rate sensors. The third-party application helps determine the medical fitness of the patient to be processed on cloud [22,23].

4.3.3 Communication Layer

The sensor patch is connected to Bluetooth of the mobile device enabling the communication between perception layer and mobile device. The Bluetooth network is preferred for short distance communication to give least delay in synchronization. The polling of data is a featured event in the physical layer to communicate the device exclusively with the gateway of the system [24].

The data aggregation is carried out at the edge device to generate the user data profile for a fixed duration of time. The sufficient data for a day is collected and processed at apache flink. The device is coordinated with a medical database system on cloud for precise streaming of the report after processing on the gateway of the perception layer in the communication. The delay in perceiving the input stream

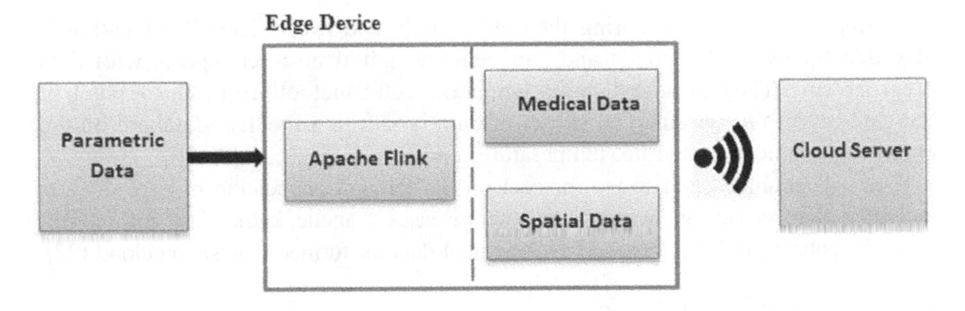

FIGURE 4.2 Communication Model for Healthcare System.

with multivalued data is minimized with Bluetooth network significantly improving the computation speed in server side training mechanism (Figure 4.2).

The data is streamed from patient to edge device with unique patient ID. The patient ID is the primary attribute to store data in the database.

Data preprocessing is a primary objective of the edge device. The streamed data with biosensor and GPS are needed to get a filter with Apache flink framework to structure the data in relevant form. The data preprocessing excludes the noise, irrelevant activity of GPS, and repetitive coordinates. Thus, it concentrates on the relevant data only for classification on cloud and hence, the edge device reduces the delay between the computing server and the end user.

4.3.4 Computing Model

The processed data is stored on the cloud with three general categories, namely behavioral data, real-time data, and medical data (Figure 4.3).

Behavioral data analysis improves the digital healthcare system in epidemic and pandemic diseases. The early detection in infectious diseases can prevent the community transmission by tracing movement of patients. The GPS and accelerometer in mobile devices can detect the activities and travelling traces of users with precise support of APIs. The particular treatment can be given to patients by

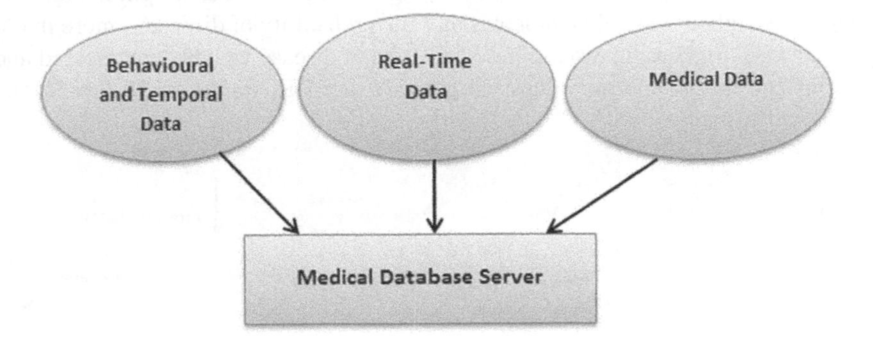

FIGURE 4.3 Three Input Medical Database System.

analyzing behavioral data during the cold, cough, and fever. The GPS location is recorded for every 3 seconds and can generate initial abstract reports with data preprocessing. The real-time data is aggregated with Bluetooth from sensor patch to the gateway of the system. The subset of data is sent to a medical database on the cloud that includes heart rate, temperature, and respiratory rate [25,26].

The patient should update the medical profile through application in edge devices including blood group, age, weight, and other diseases (diabetic, kidney function, cancer, etc). The patient profile is recorded as a medical data for further analysis on cloud [27].

4.3.4.1 Classification Model

AI provides data analytics on the pattern by learning techniques. ML techniques crack the patterns for instance input and predict the probability of occurrence of an event. The medical database system is trained with the supervised ML algorithm (Figure 4.4).

The data preprocessing is the preliminary step to filter the data set before training the model. The noise, null value, and irrelevant information are to be featured with preprocessing in the model. The success of classification in supervised learning models depends on preprocessing to feature the data set in required attributes. The further instance-based prediction is dependent on the training phase of the data model. The three class classifier is defined to intend the polled data in corresponding category to further recommend the actions for users. Input instances are streamed from edge devices for classifier with exclusive features of medical and travel history to define the precise category of patient [28,29].

The data set is referred with 500 records with 5 features. The actual data set is recorded with 150 entries with real-time approach.

The model is trained with the standard data set after preprocessing attributed in Table 4.4.

Table 4.5 shows the data attribute categories that are considered to train the model in system with behavioral, real time, and medical data.

The medical database system is trained with a data model in supervised learning form to classify the patients in three categories – Class A, Class B, and Class C – for epidemic disease with initial, moderate, and severe levels of symptoms. The classification is based on similar data valued for respective classes in the training phase.

While preparing data for processing with regard to any specific model, the certain weights are decided for parameters, e.g., for age; old age weight is high and young age weight is less. This indicates that the probability of disease is more in old age. Likewise, for chronic disease based on type of disease weights are decided and same for current parametric values temperature and HR. Based on all these, total

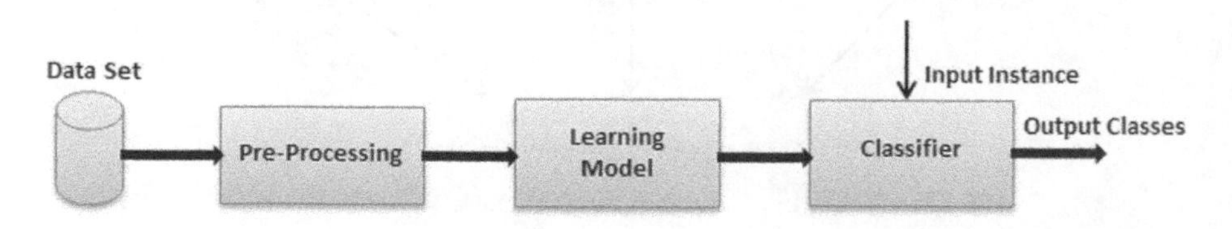

FIGURE 4.4 Supervised Learning Model.

TABLE 4.4
Parametric Data

Number	Data attribute	Remark
1	Age	Age in years
2	Gender	Male or female
3	HR	Heart rate in beats per minute(bpm_1)
4	Temp	Body temperature
5	RR	Respiratory rate in breaths per minute(bpm_2)
6	Max HR	Maximum heart rate
7	HBP	High blood pressure
8	Loc	Location with history Activity performed
9	Act	
10	Time	

weight is calculated and that provides more optimistic calculations for correctness in the system. There are two different ways to carry out this process: weighted data can be provided to the training model or training model will process the calculations considering the appropriate weights for dataset parameters.

The standard deviation with normal distribution is shown in Figure 4.5.

The area under the curve for Class A is large. The significant distribution is observed with standard deviation ±1 and around 68.27% of normal distribution is occupied. The exclusive area (excluding Class A) for Class B is relatively small with distribution of 32.82%. The rest of the area is independently upheld by Class C with least distribution but high level of pandemic symptoms.

The primary classification is featured as:

- **Class A:** The patient showing the initial symptomatic behavior towards pandemic with real-time data values. The patient can get monitored for a couple of days in the quarantine phase to avoid the panic test for pandemic. The multi-parametric real-time data HR, RR, and Temp are synchronized with threshold value.
- **Class B:** The moderate stage of symptoms, data is polled from the user for the duration of time on cloud. The patients in this class are more prone to

TABLE 4.5
Data Attribute Categories

Data Categories	Data Attribute
Behavioral and temporal	Loc, Act, Time
Real time	HR, Temp, RR, MaxHR
Medical	Age, Gender, Diab

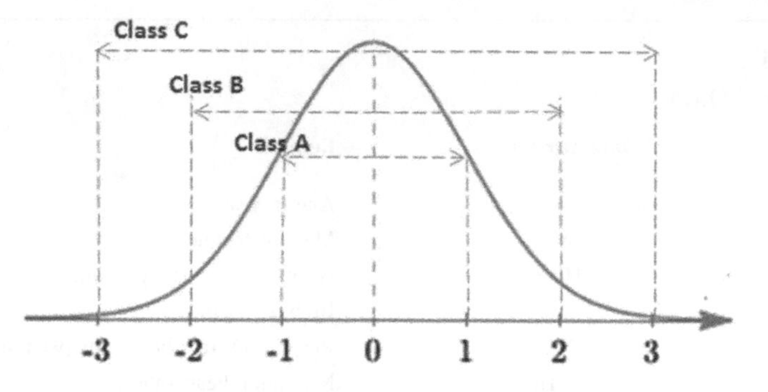

FIGURE 4.5 Parametric Standard Deviation.

infection based on the parametric values. The deviation is assumed to be large in real-time data values of patient.

- **Class C:** The deviation in data inputs HR, Temp, RR from mean value is sufficient to tag the patient in Class C. The final stage of symptoms is monitored and more prone to positive test in pandemic. The patients are recommended for testing with precautionary measures from medical authorities.

Proposed Algorithm

```
Input: HR, RR, and Temp
Output: Probabilistic Model
for (each day Time) do
Input HR, RR, Temp;
Standard Deviation (SD) HR, RR, Temp;
if (SD <= ±1)

Classify Class A;

ValidateMedical Data (age, gender, Diab), Behavioral
Data (Loc, Act)
elseif (±2 ≥ SD > ±1)

Classify Class B;

ValidateMedical Data (age, gender, Diab), Behavioral
Data (Loc, Act)
elseif (±3 ≥ SD > ±2)

Classify Class C;

ValidateMedical Data (age, gender, Diab), Behavioral
Data (Loc, Act)
End for
```

4.4 CASE STUDY: COVID-19 PANDEMIC

The proposed model is studied for COVID-19 pandemic treatment and recommendation for testing. The proposed case study highlights the need for testing with real time, behavioral, and medical data analysis. The patients are classified in classes to decide the level of severity with multivalue parameters in the medical database system.

The following severity index model for COVID-19 is proposed to classify the user in subclass as per the proposed algorithm in Section 4.3.4.1 (Figure 4.6).

The preprocessed data with behavioral, real-time, and medical records are substantial input to the classification model. The patients are sampled primarily into Class A, B, and C. The severity index is sampled into High, Moderate, and Low subclass to recommend the medical assistant to the patient. The purpose of severity index is to provide testing availability with priority and cost-effective assistant [30,31].

The taxonomy of testing is shown in Figure 4.7 with possibility of outcome of testing as True Positive, False Positive, True Negative, and False Negative. The False Positive and False Negative are the Type I and Type II errors in prediction model. The erroneous cases are small and can be monitored momentously. The probability of epidemic burst is more in case of false results. The asymptomatic patients are generally more prone to community transfer and need to be handled carefully. The large sample size is successfully categorized into True Positive and True Negative to provide the probabilistic model of testing in quarantine zone [32,33].

The low severity index is prone towards the negative test with least standard deviation. The samples in the lower curve are shown in Figure 4.8 with least severity index and designated as non-pandemic patients with preliminary symptoms and to be quarantined at home for precautionary measures.

The contagion samples are tested positive for infectious disease with symptoms based on real-time data analysis. The distribution of positive samples is shown in the upper curve in Figure 4.7. The patients under the curve are traced with location from behavioral data and are to be isolated from the community to avoid the

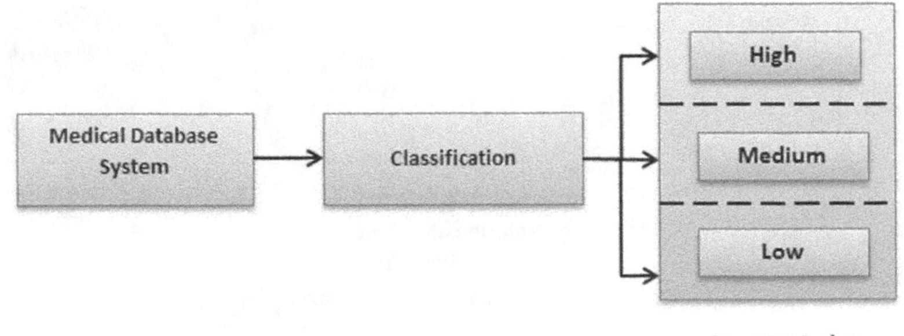

FIGURE 4.6 Severity Index Model for COVID-19.

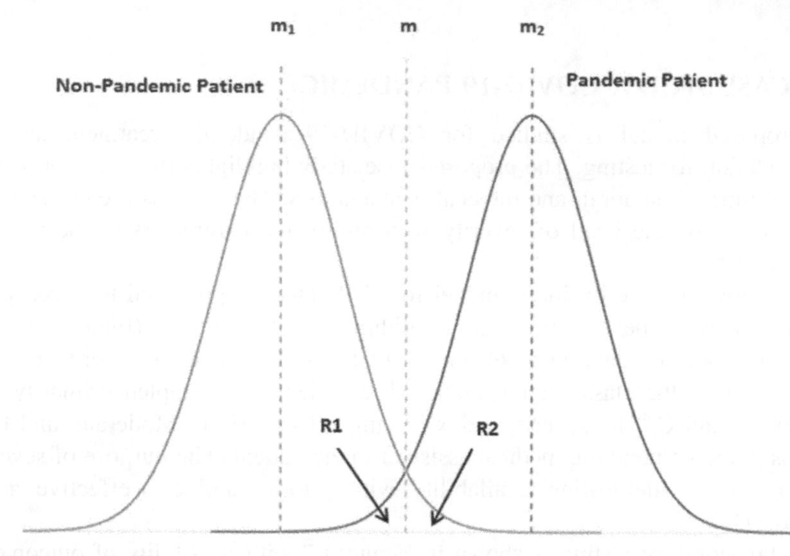

FIGURE 4.7 The Normal Distribution of Pandemic and Non-Pandemic Patient.

epidemic spread of the disease. The GPS location *loc* data attribute is processed to trace the travel history of patient.

Standard Gaussian distribution is standardized to reference. The standardization process means subtraction of inclined elements and distribution center and dividing this with standard deviation.

For medical data parameters like HR, max HR, temperature, glucose, respiration, etc., there is no fixed value but there are desirable ranges which are taken from the study of a large population and risk factors associated with parameters. Gaussian distribution or normal distribution is a bell-shaped curve, and it is assumed that measured values will follow a normal distribution. However, the value of the mean,

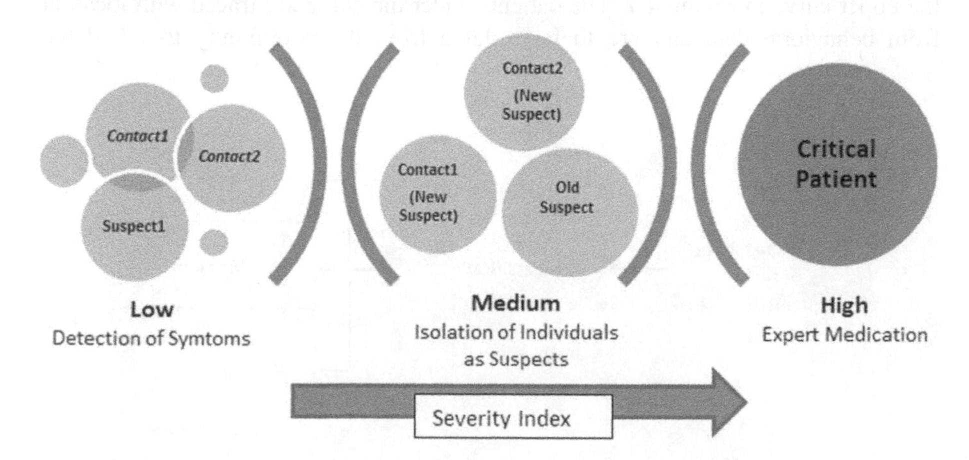

FIGURE 4.8 Phases of the Case (COVID-19).

median, and mode are varied if distribution is skewed which is not Gaussian distribution.

The mean m is the average distribution of function about the curve to define the classifications of patients. Mean m1 and m2 are the average distributions of the patient under the curve for non-pandemic and pandemic categories of samples. The region R1 shows the pandemic sample value deviated as non-pandemic (false negative) with least symptoms. The prone patients carry the infection asymptomatically and, hence, classified as a healthy sample value [34].

The region R2 (likely to be false positive) shows the higher order symptoms for disease tested negative for infection in contagion. The higher order symptoms may be prone to the positive test of the COVID-19. In both regions, confidence of samples is following characteristics of the parent curve towards peak and more prone to shift at tail. The cluster of the sample shifts to right or left depending on time function [35,36]. The patients at both the region R1 and R2 are considered as severe to pandemic and recommended for isolation from society as a precautionary measure.

If the case of COVID-19 is studied, it is observed that the disease is having its growth across time as well as space. Hence, the observatory system should follow the severity of the disease symptoms across a defined time frame. At the same time the suspect should be isolated from its neighboring contacts as shown in Figure 4.8.

The suspect of the COVID-19 needs to be tracked across the time (14-day period) and also the geographical location to find its further spread. It can be made possible by using the blockchains (Figure 4.9) that can ensure about getting live updates of the disease spread patterns to every individual involved in it. The network of the blockchain is limited to the areas declared as sensitive hotspots to overcome the limitation of blockchain towards scalability issues.

The proposed system allows symptomatic and remote data access in pandemic diseases without clinical infrastructure. The clinical, real-time, and behavioral instances of input are provided to assure the accuracy in the prediction model. The preprocessing at edge devices can enhance the precise behavior of data models towards streamed input from medical database systems on the cloud [37].

The recommendation of testing with data analysis can reduce the burden on medical infrastructure in epidemic periods. The rapid testing problem can get minimized making it financially sound.

Suggested system will help in optimizing the number of tests needed to be carried out for COVID-19 like pandemic disease. As these tests are costly and time-consuming, the system precisely suggests whether to go for the test or not. Early or unnecessary tests may create panic situations among society, which can be avoided by use of a suggested system.

One of the basic advantages of the system is; with the minor modifications in consultation with medical experts, the system can be configured for new disease detection.

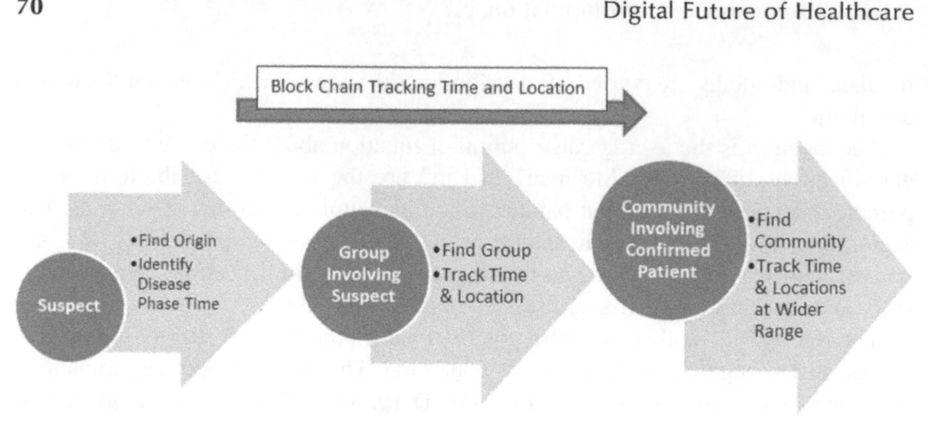

FIGURE 4.9 Track of the Case (COVID-19).

4.5 LIMITATIONS AND FUTURE SCOPE

The proposed model is based on symptomatic behavior of the human body with data fetched from biosensors. The model is unable to predict the state of the patient in asymptomatic behavior and, hence, having the possibility of false negative predictions (Figure 4.10).

Similarly, the higher order symptoms with real-time data values are predicted with false positive cases. The false prediction models are to be trained separately with data sets. The error model with additional parametric values is to be considered in processing the data at the server side.

The probabilistic model with iterative training is to be proposed to reduce the error in the prediction model. The iterative training with more parametric values can improve the performance of the system. The multi-sensor attributes with incremental epoch may reduce the false prediction. The virtual container-based data processing can compute huge data with least delay in epoch-based computation. The potential of a system can be enhanced with distributed computing in big data processing. The coverage of edge devices and biosensors can be empowered with

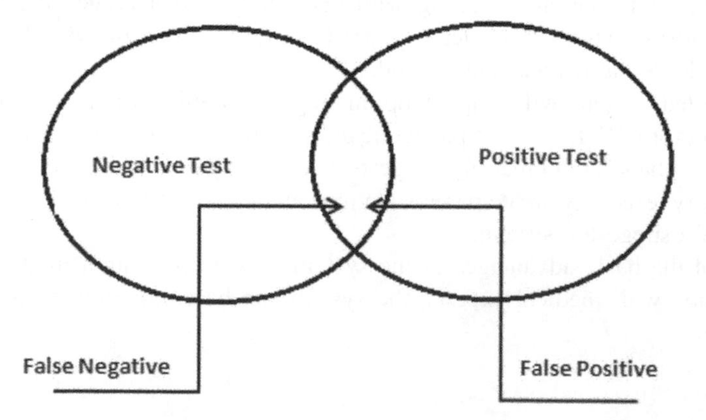

FIGURE 4.10 Type I and Type II Error in Prediction Model.

nodal computation in distributed cloud-based systems. Distributed cloud processing can improve the computation power with a multi-epoch environment. The virtual platform will scale the volume of computation to provide reliable and fast decision-making in ML.

REFERENCES

1. Hyun Jung La, Han Ter Jung, Soo Dong Kim, "Extensible Disease Diagnosis Cloud Platform with Medical Sensors and IoT Devices", *3rd International Conference on Future Internet of Things and Cloud*, ISBN: 978-1-4673-8103-1, 2015.
2. Y. Li, C. He, X. Fan, X Huang, Y. Cai, O. Terzo, L. Mossucca, "HCloud a Healthcare-Oriented Cloud System with Improved Efficiency in Biomedical Data Processing", In *Cloud Computing with e-Science Applications*. USA: CRC Press, pp. 164–190, 2015.
3. Dineshkumar, R. SenthilKumar, K. Sujatha, R.S. Ponmagal, "Big Data Analytics of IoT Based Health Care Monitoring System", *IEEE Uttar Pradesh Section International Conference on Electrical, Computer and Electronics Engineering (UPCON)*, ISSN:978-1-5090-5384-1, 2016.
4. Ahmed Dridi, Salma Sassi, Sami Faiz, "A Smart Platform for Personalized Healthcare Monitoring Using Semantic Technologies", *IEEE 29th International Conference on Tools with Artificial Intelligence (ICTAI)*, pp. 393–398, 2017.
5. Kavita Jaiswal, Debasish Jena, Bibhudatta SahooL, "An IoT-Cloud Based Smart Healthcare Monitoring System Using Container Based Virtual Environment in Edge Device", *International Conference on Emerging Trends and Innovations in Engineering and Technological Research (ICETIETR)*, pp. 2679–2687, 2018.
6. Iman Azimi, Janne Takalo-Mattila, Arman Anzanpour, Amir M. Rahmani, Juha-Pekka Soininen, Pasi Liljeb, "Empowering Healthcare IoT Systems with Hierarchical Edge-Based Deep Learning", *IEEE/ACM International Conference on Connected Health: Applications, Systems and Engineering Technologies(CHASE)*, ISBN 978-1-4503-5958-0, 2018.
7. Inderpreet Singh, Deepak Kumar, Sunil Kumar Khatri, "Improving the Efficiency of E-Healthcare System Based on Cloud", *Amity International Conference on Artificial Intelligence (AICAI)*, ISBN: 978-1-5386-9346-9, 2019.
8. Sherali Zeadally, Farhan Siddiqui, Zubair Baig, Ahmed Ibrahim, "Challenges and Potential Solutions Using Internet of Things (IoT) and Big Data Analytics", *PSU Research Review*, vol. 4, no. 2, pp. 1494–1516, 2019.
9. Asaph Azaria, Ariel Ekblaw, Thiago Vieira, Andrew Lippman, "A Case Study for Blockchain in Healthcare: Prototype for Electronic Health Records and Medical Research Data", *MedRec Publication*, vol. 2, pp. 133–138, 2016.
10. Vidhya Ramani, Tanesh Kumar, An Bracken, Madhusanka Liyanage, Mika Ylianttila, "Secure and Efficient Data Accessibility in Blockchain Based Healthcare Systems", *IEEE Global Communications Conference (GLOBECOM)*, ISSN: 2576-6813, 2018.
11. Anuraag A. Vazirani, Odhran O'Donoghue, David Brindley, "Implementing Blockchains for Efficient Health Care: Systematic Review", *Journal of Medical Internet Research*, vol. 21, no. 2, ISBN 2278-1021, pp. e12439, 2019.
12. Kwame Omono Asamoah, Jianbin Gao, "MeDShare: Trust-less Medical Data Sharing Among Cloud Service Providers Via Blockchain", *IEEE Access*, vol. 5, no. 3, ISSN: 2169-3536, pp. 14757–14767, 2019.
13. Leila Ismail, Huned Materwala, Sherali Zeadally, "Lightweight Blockchain for Healthcare", *IEEE Access*, vol. 7, pp. 1611–1618, 2019.

14. Anton Hasselgrena, Katina Kralevskab, Danilo Gligoroskib, Sindre A. Pedersenc, Arild Faxvaag, "Blockchain in Healthcare and Health Sciences—A Scoping Review", *International Journal of Medical Informatics*, vol. 134, pp. 124–130, 2020.
15. Niharika G. Maity, Sreerupa Das, "Machine Learning for Improved Diagnosis and Prognosis in Healthcare", *IEEE Aerospace Conference*, pp. 210–228, 2017.
16. Shubham Jayawant, "Medic: An Artificially Intelligent System to Provide Healthcare Services to Society and Medical Assistance to Doctors", *International Conference on Communication and Electronics Systems (ICCES)*, ISBN: 978-1-5090-1066-0, 2017.
17. M. Callejon, D. Naranjo, J. Reina-Tosina, L. Roa, "Distributed Circuit Modeling of Galvanic and Capacitive Coupling for Intrabody Communication", *IEEE Transactions on Biomedical Engineering*, vol. 59, no. 11, pp. 3263–3269, 2012.
18. Ria Maheshwari, Kartik Moudgil, Harshal Parekh, Rupali Sawant, "A Machine Learning Based Medical Data Analytics and Visualization Research Platform", *IEEE Conference on Communication and Electronics Systems*, ISBN: 978-1-5090-1066-0, 2018.
19. Muhammad Azeem Sarwar, Nasir Kamal, Wajeeha Hamid, Munam Ali Shah, "Prediction of Diabetes Using Machine Learning Algorithms in Healthcare", *24th International Conference on Automation and Computing (ICAC)*, ISSN: 1159-2536, 2018.
20. Tran Le Nguyen, Thi Thu Ha Do, "Artificial Intelligence in Healthcare to Train the Patient Before Surgery", *Portland International Conference on Management of Engineering and Technology (PICMET)*, ISSN: 2159-5100, 2013.
21. Syed Umar Amin, M. Shamim Hossain, "Cognitive Smart Healthcare for Pathology Detection and Monitoring", *IEEE Access*, vol. 6, pp. 40846–40853, 2019.
22. D. Antolin, N. Medrano, B. Calvo, F. Pérez, "A Wearable Wireless Sensor Network for Indoor Smart Environment Monitoring in Safety Applications", *Sensors MDPI*, vol. 17, no. 2, pp. 365, 2017.
23. H. R. Roth, Le Lu, Jiamin Liu, Jianhua Yao, Ari Seff, Kevin Cherry, Lauren Kim, Ronald M. Summers, "Improving Computer-Aided Detection Using Convolutional Neural Networks and Random View Aggregation", *IEEE Transactions on Medical Imaging*, vol. 35, no. 5, pp. 1170–1181, May, 2016.
24. Sunil Tamhankar, Shefali Sonavane, Mayur Rathi, Faruk Kazi, "Smart Sensing of Medical Disorder Detection for Physically Impaired Person", *Science Direct Academic Press*, pp. 179–200, 2020.
25. Nilanjan Dey, Aboul EllaHassanien, Chintan Bhatt, Amira S Ashour, Suresh Chandra Satapathy, *Internet of Things and Big Data Analytics Toward Next-Generation Intelligence*. Berlin: Springer, pp. 3–549, 2018.
26. Md. Golam Sarowar, Md. Sarwar Kamal, Nilanjan Dey, *Internet of Things and Its Impacts in Computing Intelligence: A Comprehensive Review – IoT Application for Big Data*. USA: IGI Global, pp. 103–136, 2019.
27. R. Fakoor, F. Ladhak, A. Nazi, M. Huber, "Using Deep Learning to Enhance Cancer Diagnosis and Classification", *Proceedings of the International Conference on Machine Learning*, pp. 1–7, 2013.
28. Teresa Piliouras, Xin Tian, Dhaval Desai, Avani Patel, Dhara Shah, Yang Su, Pui Lam Yu, Nadia Sultana, "Impacts of Legislation on Electronic Health Records Systems and Security Implementation", *Systems, Applications and Technology Conference (LISAT) IEEE Long Island*, pp. 1–7, 2012.
29. M. Vida, O. Lupse, L. Stoicu-Tivadar, "Improving the Interoperability of Healthcare Information Systems Through HL& CDA and CCD Standards", *7th IEEE*

International Symposium on Applied Computational Intelligence and Informatics. Timisoara, Romania, pp. 157–161, 2012.

30. T. Namli, G. Aluc, A. Dogac, "An Interoperability Test Framework for HL7-Based Systems", *IEEE Transactions on Information Technology in Biomedicine*, vol. 13, no. 3, pp. 389–399, May, 2009.
31. N. Kabra, A. Nadkarni, "Prevalence of Depression and Anxiety in Irritable Bowel Syndrome: A Clinic Based Study from India", *Indian Journal of Psychiatry*, vol. 55, no. 1, pp. 77, 2013.
32. Arkaprabha Sau, Ishita Bhakta, "Predicting Anxiety and Depression in Elderly Patients Using Machine Learning Technology", *Healthcare Technology Letters*, vol. 4, ISSN: 2053-3713, 2017.
33. A.-M. Rahmani, N. K. Thanigaivelan, T. N. Gia, J. Granados, B. Negash, P. Liljeberg, H. Tenhunen, "Smart E-health Gateway: Bringing Intelligence to Internet-of-Things Based Ubiquitous Healthcare Systems", *12th Annual IEEE Consumer Communications and Networking Conference* (CCNC), pp. 826–834, 2015.
34. F. Bonomi, R. Milito, J. Zhu, S. Addepalli, "Fog Computing and Its Role in the Internet of Things", *Proceedings of the First Edition of the MCC Workshop on Mobile Cloud Computing*, pp. 13–16, 2012.
35. I. Stojmenovic, S. Wen, "The Fog Computing Paradigm: Scenarios and Security Issues", *Federated Conference on Computer Science and Information Systems (FedCSIS)*, pp. 1–8, 2014.
36. C. He, X. Fan, Y. Li, "Toward Ubiquitous Healthcare Services with a Novel Efficient Cloud Platform", *IEEE Transactions on Biomedical Engineering*, vol. 60, no. 1, pp. 230–234, 2013.
37. G. Suciu, V. Suciu, A. Martian, R. Craciunescu, A. Vulpe, I. Marcu, S. Halunga, O. Fratu, "Big Data Internet of Things and Cloud Convergence-An Architecture for Secure E-health Applications", *Journal of Medical Systems*, vol. 39, no. 11, pp. 1–8, 2015.

5 Epileptic Aura Detection to Rescue the Epilepsy Patient Through Wireless Body Area Sensor Network

Alo Sen[1], Ratula Ray[2], Rahul Roy[1], and Satya Ranjan Dash[2]
[1]ei2 Classes and Technologies, Durgapur, West Bengal, India
[2]Kalinga Institute of Industrial Technology, Deemed to be University, Bhubaneswar, India

CONTENTS

5.1 INTRODUCTION

5.1.1 EPILEPSY ATTACK

Epilepsy is the most common neurological disorder that can affect anyone at any age. It is a chronic disorder in which brain activities become abnormal. Epilepsy is "a

DOI: 10.1201/9781003198796-5

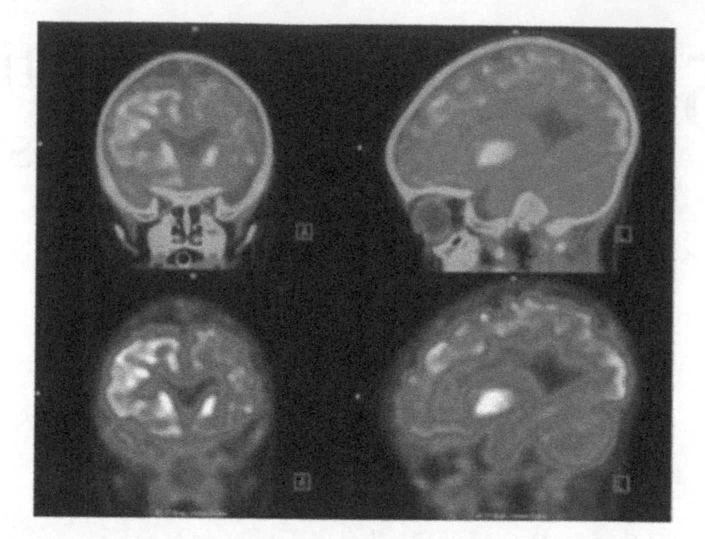

FIGURE 5.1 Epilepsy Attack in Human Brain.

common neurological condition characterized by recurrent seizures." Figure 5.1 shows an epilepsy attack in brain [1]. One-third of the people with epilepsy exist with unmanageable seizers due to lack of treatment. Whereas six out of ten cases of epilepsy in individuals is unidentified. Around 150,000 new cases of epilepsy are reported in the United States each year. Repeated seizures are the main symptom of epilepsy.

Some of the symptoms include convulsion with no fever, unresponsive to instructions, falls without any reason, sudden bouts of chewing, blinking with no reason, changes in senses like smell, sound, and touch, sudden fear in mind, panic, etc. A person is affected by an epilepsy attack when the messaging system is interrupted by faulty electrical activity in the brain. Some people get epilepsy attack due to inherited genetic factors. Many other factors are stroke or tumor, AIDS, brain damage that occurs before birth, viral encephalitis, autism, or neurofibromatosis. The World Health Organization (WHO) stated that approximately 50 million people are affected by epilepsy in the world. About 1.2% of the U.S. population, or 3 million adults and 470,000 children, suffered from an epilepsy attack. Idiopathic, cryptogenic, and symptomatic are the three types of epileptic seizures that can occur in a patient. There is no specific reason for the first case, in the second case the actual reason for the attack cannot be found easily, and in the third case the actual cause of the attack can be found out easily. Table 5.1 illustrates the different types of seizures which indicate the part of brain where the seizure activity started (Table 5.2).

TABLE 5.1
Variety in Partial Seizure

Simple partial seizure	Complex partial seizure
• Patient remain conscious • Being aware of surroundings	• Patient's consciousness is impaired • He cannot remember the attack

TABLE 5.2
Variety in Generalized Seizure

Tonic-clonic seizure	• Body stiffness • Shaking • Loss of consciousness
Absence seizure	• Patient undergo short lapses in consciousness
Tonic seizure	• Patient may fall due to stiffness of muscle
Atonic seizure	• Patient fall suddenly due to loss of muscle control
Clonic seizure	• Rhythmic jerking movement of patient

Secondary generalized seizure: This type of attack starts as a partial seizure but spreads into the whole brain. In severe cases, the patient loses consciousness.

5.1.2 Body Area Network

A body area network (BAN) is also popularly known as wireless body area network (WBAN). It is generally a computing device which is wearable. BAN consists of different types of biomedical sensors and gateway like normal mobile phones and smart mobile phones. The mobile phone should have an Internet connection through either 3G/4G wireless or Wi-Fi. The data that get collected by the sensor finally gets delivered to remote server or cloud. Figure 5.2 illustrates a typical BAN connected to a patient [2].

BAN architecture consists of three levels communications.

1. **Intra-BAN Level:** In this layer, communication between the master node and the body sensors takes place.
2. **Inter-BAN Level:** In this layer, communication takes place between the master node and personal devices such as notebooks and home service robots.
3. **Beyond-BAN Level:** It connects the personal device to the Internet and Figure 5.3 illustrates general architecture of BAN [3].

5.1.2.1 Technologies Associated with BAN

1. Bluetooth
2. Bluetooth Low Energy (BLE)
3. Zigbee and 802.15.4
4. IEEE 802.11
5. IEEE 802.15.6
6. Ultra Wideband (UWB)
7. ANT Protocol [4]
8. The Zarlink Technology [5,6]
9. Rubee active wireless protocol [6,7]

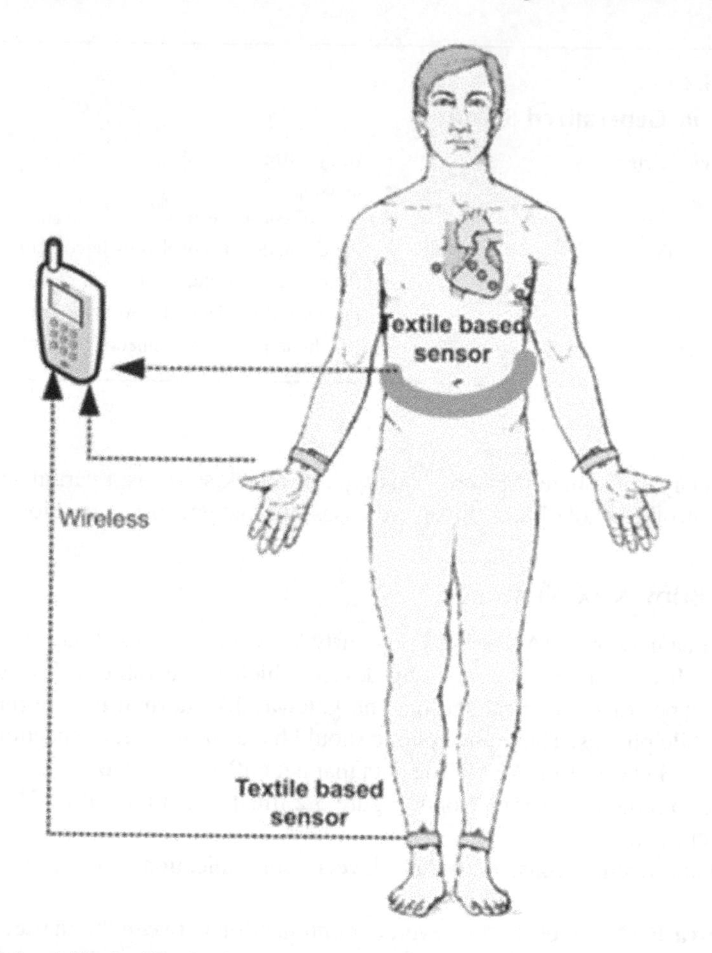

FIGURE 5.2 A Typical Body Area Network Connected to a Patient.

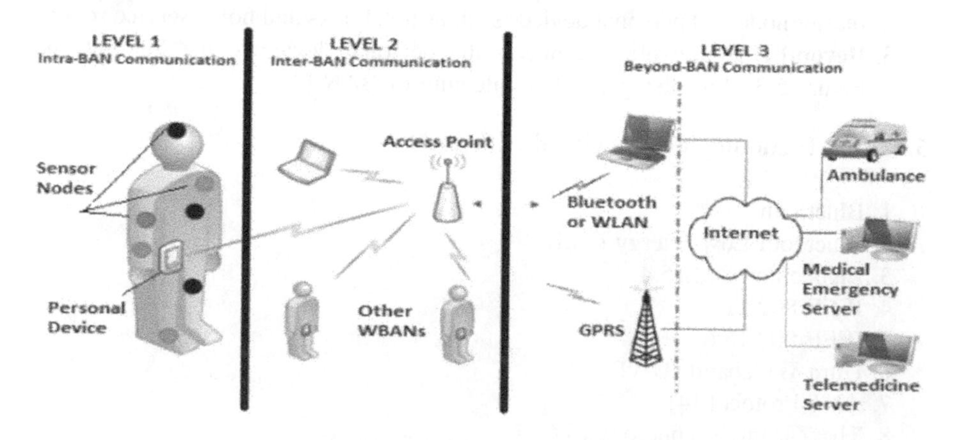

FIGURE 5.3 General Architecture of BAN.

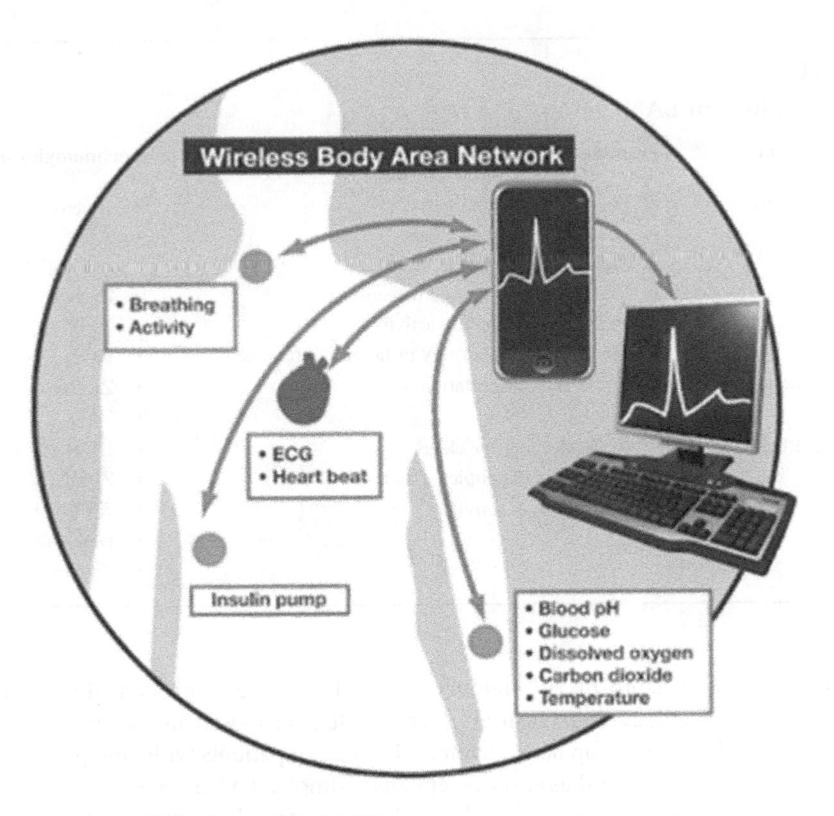

FIGURE 5.4 Working Principle of BAN.

BAN adds a new era in medical science. It has many proven applications in different medical healthcare problems. Figure 5.4 illustrates different areas where BAN has provided great results.

Table 5.3 describes various applications of BAN with associated technology.

5.2 RELATED WORK

Literature survey showed the use of a fully automated algorithm with minimum human interaction. Due to close resemblance with the features associated with an epileptic spike, eye blink is often considered as a confusing form of artifact. The study suggests the use of an unsupervised method for removing eye blink artifacts via Discrete Wavelet Transform (DWT) by using Bior 3.3. Within a duration of 23.6 seconds, the paper shows the use of 200 EEG signals and 4,097 sample points for each case (100 signals from healthy subjects and 100 for epileptic subjects, respectively). For each signal, 16 windows have been segmented and the noisy signals were discarded. The DWT coefficients were isolated using Db4 mother wavelet for three levels (eye blink artifact removal using DWT, extraction of features, and classification) and statistical features for all four sub-bands were calculated. The suggested approach showed improved results upon the performance of

TABLE 5.3
Applications of BAN

Application	Examples	Technologies used
Telemedecine	• Health monitor remotely • Rescue in emergency case • Monitoring of chronic diseases • Disease prevention and detection • Monitoring of routine activity • Monitoring post-surgery in-home improvement	• Bluetooth • ANT • IEEE 802.15.6 • ZigBee • WiFi • RFID
Rehabilitation	Daily life and rehabilitation	• ZigBee • WiFi
Assisted living	• Assisted living for elders • Treatments of peoples at home	• IEEE 802.15.6 • ZigBee
Biofeedback	User biofeedback activity	• ANT • Bluetooth • ZigBee

ANFIS (adaptive neuro-fuzzy inference system) classifier with considerable improvement in accuracy and sensitivity. The system proposed in the paper shows great potential and opens up newer avenues in treating patients with epilepsy, which can save time and make diagnosis of epilepsy simpler and more efficient. As an early stage detection system of epilepsy for presurgical evaluation, the abovementioned system can be highly effective.

For detection of epileptic seizures by intrinsic mode functions (IMF) and extraction of features by Empirical Mode Decomposition (EMD) method, study [8] suggests a layout for carrying out the work. Using the database of the Epileptology Department of Bonn University for the purpose of the study, the classification task was being conducted. The dataset comprised five marker groups where records of healthy persons and patients with epilepsy had been decomposed into IMFs by using the EMD method. The feature vectors were being extracted based on Tsallis, Renyi, and Relative Entropy and Coherence approaches. After the completion of the extraction processes, the classification task was carried out by Naive Bayes Classifier (NBC), K-Nearest Neighbors Classifier (KNN), and Linear Discriminant Analysis (LDA).

Assessment for the relative epileptogenic potential in neuronal systems that are of bi-stable nature has been done in study [9]. Based on the use of an active probing paradigm that involves stimulation of the system with pulses of increasing amplitudes, the method is used for automatic detection of signs of approaching the transition point regarding intensity of stimulation, without allowing the actual seizure transition to occur. The practical applicability of this method is huge and if it can be successfully applied in the clinic, the approach may create a safer option for presurgical diagnostics, which will consequently improve the quality of life of patients and caregivers. Featuring the coexistence of "normal" and oscillatory states, the authors propose a simple bi-stable model. Other than the proposed model, literature survey shows the presence of models with similar features [10,11]. The study has a potential for bringing the system closer to a biological reality which might lead to higher degree of universal acceptance of the results obtained.

The authors in this study [12] have aimed at quantifying the connector hub abnormalities in mTLE (mesial temporal lobe epilepsy) and have attempted for identifying the resting state networks of epilepsy involved in abnormal connector hubs. Disruption and emergence of all connector hubs is quantified for each of the epileptic patients and assessment of the conversion of network via connector hubs have been carried out. In case of mTLE, pathological disruption has been noticed at the basic connector hubs in the mesial temporal lobe and including default mode network. Accuracy of new connector hubs has been identified in right mTLE than for left mTLE. Survey also suggests the difference in patterns of conversion of the desired network were found in right and left mTLE of the abnormal hippocampus. Various factors such as temporal and cerebellar mode, default mode contribute to the conversion of hippocampal networks. The authors lastly reorganized a non-similar connector hub and regularized the resting state networks of mTLE in case of epilepsy. Characterization by local connections emerged and the disturbance of distant connections (arise in case if) were also carried out.

Depending upon the accelerometer for the detection of epileptic seizure, the study [13] also proposes an effective seizure detection system. A wireless sensor network (WSN) was created, which was aimed at improving the life of patients.

The model comprised two-dimensional accelerometer sensors placed on the right and left hand, and on left thigh, respectively, for the patient with epilepsy under study. For the development of an automatic epilepsy detection algorithm, data has been collected for three persons those suffering with severe epilepsy. WSNs have been used to locate the place of a patient in case of an emergency on detection of a seizure attack. The data collected from the sensors then were used for sending an emergency alarm to the doctor, nurse, and to the patient's parties. MICAz Motes developed by Crossbow Technology was used as the wireless sensor node for the study. The above model can find its application in cases of patients who require assisted living. The data collected were being analyzed using deep learning models such as Artificial Neural Network and normal classifiers such as KNN to recognize the difference between the normal as well as seizure movements. According to the results, KNN algorithm gives better performance than Artificial Neural Network for detection of the seizures. Finally, the result for accurate detection of epilepsy occurred only if in the total collected signal, minimum 50% of signal is seizure one. Additional advantage for this study also includes the fact that for each new patient, the algorithm need not be trained each time.

Another study [14] also included the representation of a behavioral model on physiological facts and disorder or confusion of epilepsy. The system identifies the cause and effects of abnormal seizure, and also figures out the general causes of epilepsy attack. The study also suggested that the model showed the possibility of a reciprocal action between the role of excitation and restrain neurotransmitters with regard to epilepsy. The outcome of the authors approach obtained might provide some helpful insights into fetching different causes of epilepsy and providing efficient useful guide for prediction of seizure occurrence in patients. The results obtained from the study also helps us gain detailed possibilities of epilepsy and help in the development of new prediction methods with algorithm to detect abnormal seizure attack in epilepsy patients.

Study [15] presented a hypothesis that patients with TLE (temporal lobe epilepsy) show abnormality in the homogenous functioning of the DMN (Default Mode Network), which correlate the parameters such as duration of illness, seizure age, and RT. The authors found several limitations on previous studies. First, correlation between abnormal NH and the memory cannot be established as in the previous studies, the authors had not tested the memory. Second, TLE symptomatic patients were categorized into two groups – left and right. In case of medically stable patients, the number of used AEDs, factor of AEDs and which AEDs is used are not inclined by the previous authors. The researchers focused on the DMN pathophysiologic contribution neglecting other brain region information and on the substitute in DMN. The above paper resulted in the existing patient with TLE and the abnormalities of NH of DMN. To explore NH by an accurate way to improve the nature of forwarded TLE also be understood. The above paper highlighted TLE pathophysiology with the importance of DMN.

In [16], The authors proceeded with verbal fluency behavioral measure and an fMRI verbal fluency paradigm to check with 19 healthy patients and 37 TLE patients. The data revealed that the task-driven activity pattern is not seen in the network in TLE. After observing the whole association of simple structure–function, the authors suggested that an important contribution to the impairment of cognitive analysis of epilepsy is the flexibility failure due to network.

In [17], the authors analyzed the dynamic functional network connectivity (dFNC) of all the functional systems in FLE with the pattern of temporal and spatial domains. From 19 FLE patients and 18 controls, the required fMRI resting-state data were collected. To divide RSNs, the analysis of independent component was used by grouping them in seven functional modules. The dFNC patterns were identified by sliding windows and clustering method. After that, evaluation of dynamic functional state interactions (dFSIs) and state-specific connectivity pattern were done.

In [18], the authors tried to combine the network of EEG and analysis of clustering together with variable bands of frequencies. Thus, the authors tried to monitor the activity of brain by interictal to preictal states of brain having a seizure. The authors have used k-medoids clustering approach for their study to compare the preictal state with interictal state. They observed an increase in the EEG network connectivity synchronization. The finding facts helped the successive authors for their future study to predict epileptic seizures.

In [19], the authors considered electrocardiography (ECoG) signals of 11 refractory epilepsy patients. Then the authors calculated the phase synchronization of the ECoG signals and thus established the brain network. No major difference was found in the various network transition states in the period before seizure, during seizure, and after seizure and a level of increase in the synchronization was found prior to seizure termination. The final result indicates that the transition of network state will not dominate the seizure and at the time of seizure termination, synchronization might take place.

In [20], the authors studied the influence of connections on seizures. The authors used a model which was of a simple network, comprising four neuronal populations which were interconnected. Model simulation was used to study the surgery effect on the rate of seizure. It was identified that, for the most of the cases, removal of hyper excitable population was not the best approach for the reduction of the rate of seizures. For reduction, removal of normal populations was found to be more effective at a vital spot in the network. The method of work identified that the structure of network and its connections were most important rather than finding the node of pathology.

In [21], the authors proposed ECoG system which is portable and wireless. To collect the brain activities in form of electrical signals and stimulate the suffered organ or tissue, researchers focused on an array of high resolution 32 channel ECG electrode. The proposed wireless communication circuit designed by using Bluetooth Low Energy 4 (LTE4) with cellular technology for transmission, acquisition, and processing of data. The medical test performed on living organism (in this study rat) shows that brain activities in the form of electrical signals can be recorded accurately and transmitted with a maximal sampling rate of 30 ksampling/s per channel by the flexible ECoG system. It demonstrates that the detection of epilepsy-suffered organ or tissue, exact location of suffering, and ideal treatment can be found by the ECoG system. The proposed system with low energy consumption and high brain spatial resolution was found to have great potential applications.

In [22], the authors considered all subtypes with focal seizure of 38 patients and 21 healthy controls that undergo assessment of structural MRI, neurological state, and IQ. The thickness of cortex was derived using a brain imaging software – FreeSurfer – from the structural MRIs. Subsequently, correlations of thickness of cortex were constructed in a group level by SCNs. By add-one-patient approach, the data of individual SCNs of the epilepsy patient have been extracted and added to the control group. The network measures like path length, coefficient of clustering, and centrality of betweenness of severity of epilepsy including seizure history and onset age were calculated. The result showed that the correlations between interregional variations of cortical thickness reflect disease characteristics or responses to the disease and deficits in patients with epilepsy with focal seizures.

5.3 OUR APPROACH

We have proposed three models for detection of any abnormal activity of brain to detect epilepsy attack as early as possible. Our approaches are: Close Circuit Seizer Detection, Neck Choker, and Heart Beat Sensor. Section 5.3.1 illustrates the Close Circuit Seizer Detection method. Section 5.3.2 illustrates the Neck Choker, and Section 5.3.3 illustrates seizure detection with the Heart Beat Sensor.

5.3.1 Proposed Model 1 – Close Circuit Seizure Detector

In our first model, continuous body movement of a person will be monitored by a smartphone whose camera will act as a video feeder by installing At Home Monitor App. Another smartphone can stream the video from any location by installing At Home Monitor App. Figure 5.5 shows the block diagram of Close Circuit Seizure Detector.

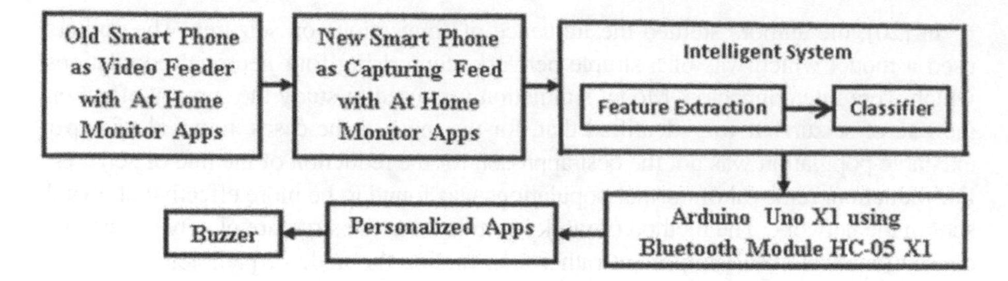

FIGURE 5.5 Block Diagram of Close Circuit Seizure Detector.

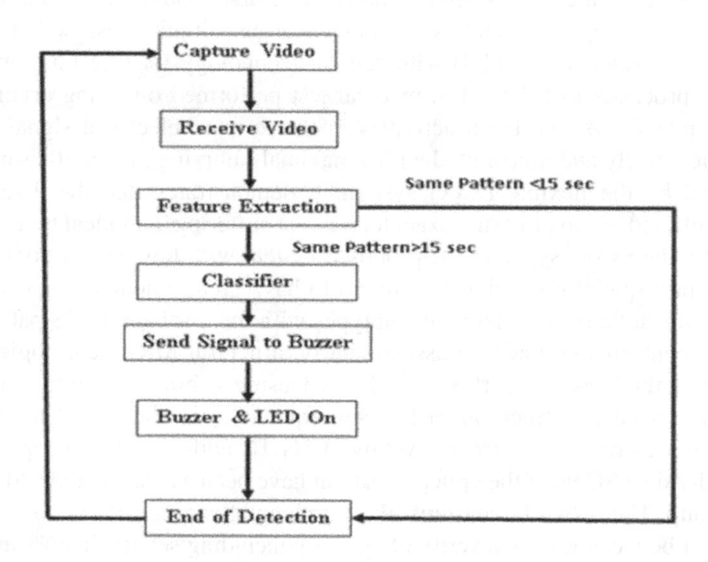

FIGURE 5.6 Workflow Diagram of Close Circuit Seizure Detector.

5.3.1.1 Initial Setup

Launch at Home Monitor App on both phones. When it is online, the app generates CID with the help of user name and password. Enter the information and it is ready to monitor the feed. Figure 5.6 shows the workflow diagram of Close Circuit Seizure Detector. The video will be sent to an intelligent system where the movement of body parts will be processed. If same pattern movement repeats for less than 15 seconds then the classifier will treat it as normal behavior otherwise it will classify the pattern of movement as abnormal. Then, it will forward a signal to the Arduino Uno XI and finally it will send the alert to the guardian by enabling the buzzer.

5.3.2 Proposed Model 2 – Neck Choker

In our second approach, one Neck Choker will be embedded with EEG module, an expert system, and one GSM module. Figure 5.7 shows the circuit diagram of EEG module. Figures 5.8–5.10 show the components of circuit diagram in bigger format

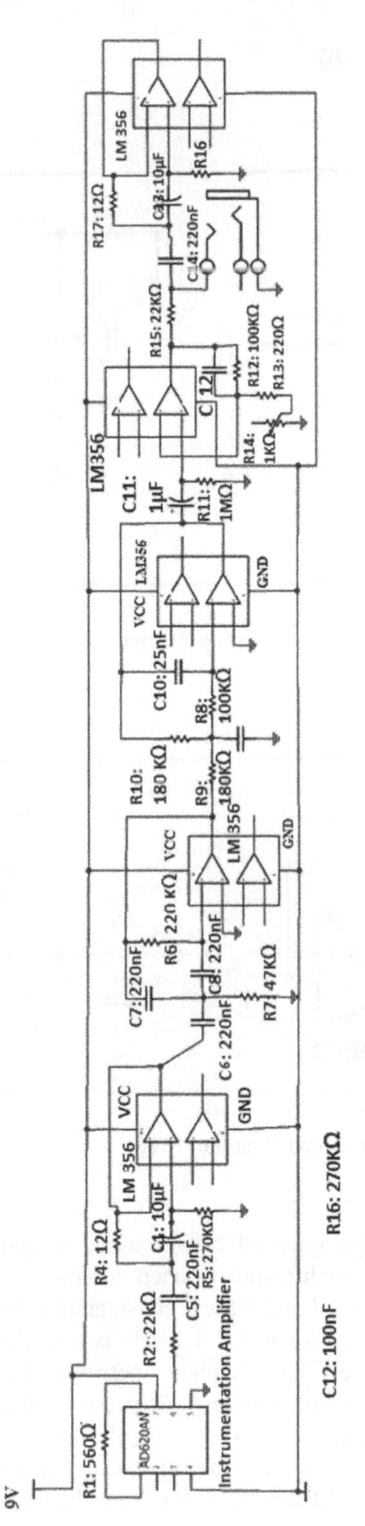

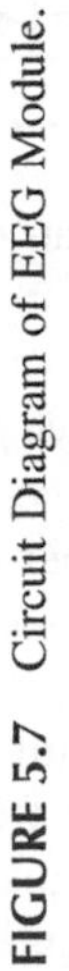
FIGURE 5.7 Circuit Diagram of EEG Module.

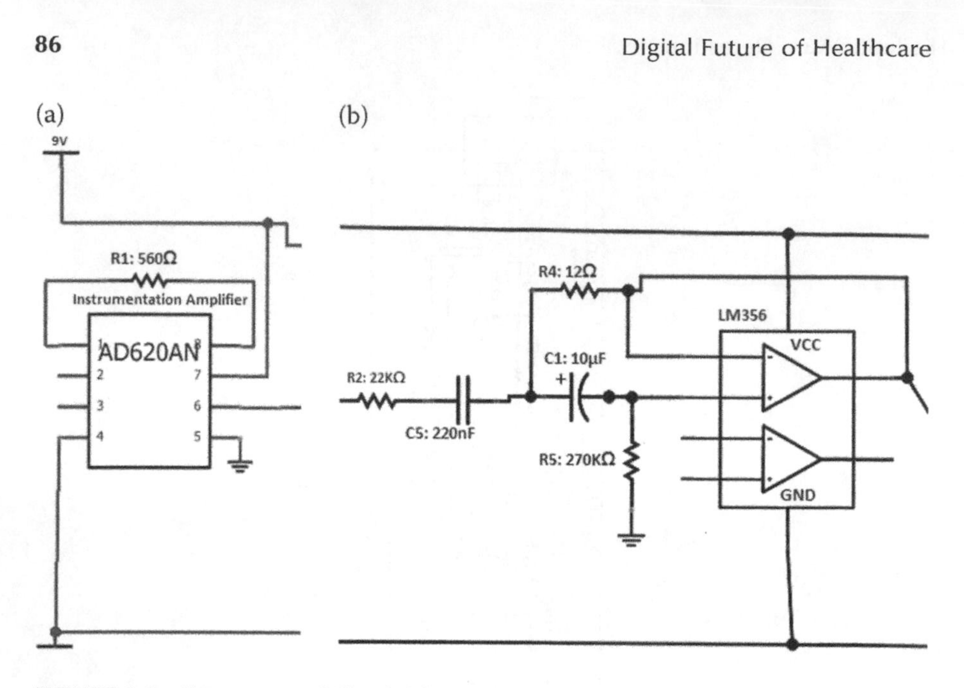

FIGURE 5.8 Components of Circuit Diagram (Bigger View). (a) Instrumentation Amplifier, (b) Notch Filter.

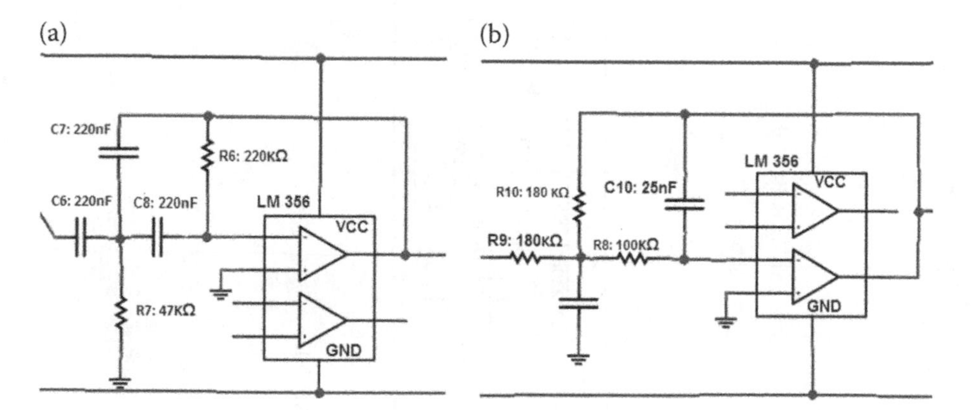

FIGURE 5.9 Components of Circuit Diagram (Bigger View). (a) 7 Hz High Pass Filter, (b) 31 Hz Low Pass Filter.

[23]. Figure 5.11 shows five types of brain waves. Frequency less than 4 Hz is considered as delta wave, which results in deep dreamless sleep with loss of body awareness, frequency between 4 and 7 Hz is considered as theta wave that results in deep meditation, frequency between 7 and 13 Hz is considered as alpha wave that results in calm relaxed yet alert state, frequency between 13 and 39 Hz is considered as beta wave which results in busy thinking, active processing, active concentration, arousal, cognition, and frequency between 40 and 50 Hz is considered as gamma wave that results in higher mental activity, including perception, problem solving, and consciousness. Figure 5.12 illustrates the flow diagram of detecting epileptic

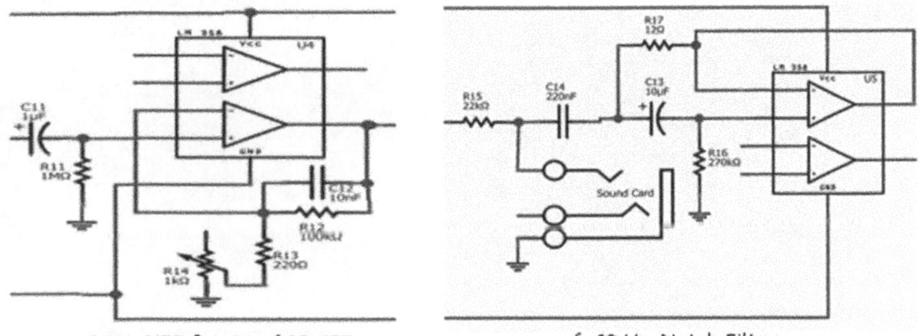

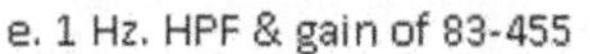

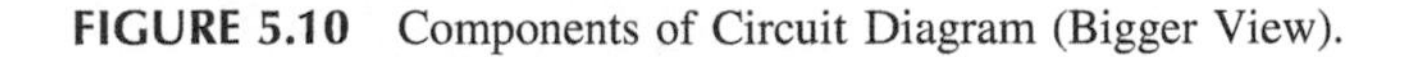
FIGURE 5.10 Components of Circuit Diagram (Bigger View).

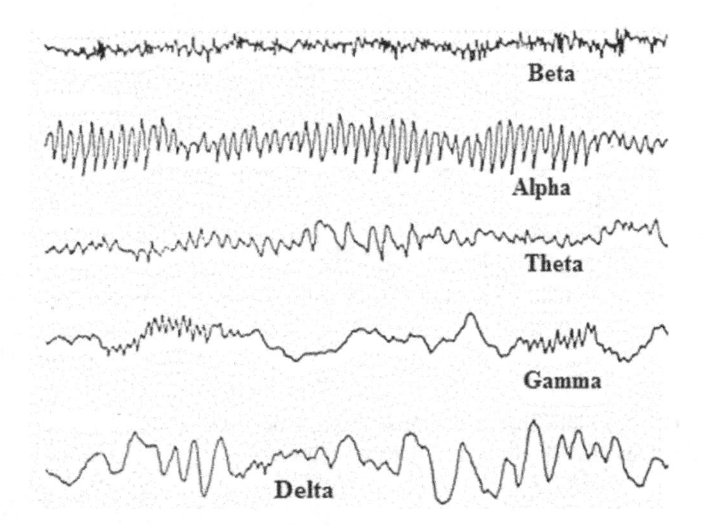

FIGURE 5.11 Five Types of Brain Waves.

signal in our proposed model. Figure 5.13 illustrates the block diagram of the working principle of the Neck Choker.

5.3.2.1 Components of EEG Module

1. 1 Pcs AD620AN
2. Capacitors
   a. 10 nF – 1 Pcs
   b. 20 nF – 1 Pcs
   c. 100 nF – 1 Pcs
   d. 220 nF – 5 Pcs
   e. 1 μF – 1 Pcs
   f. μF – 1 Pcs

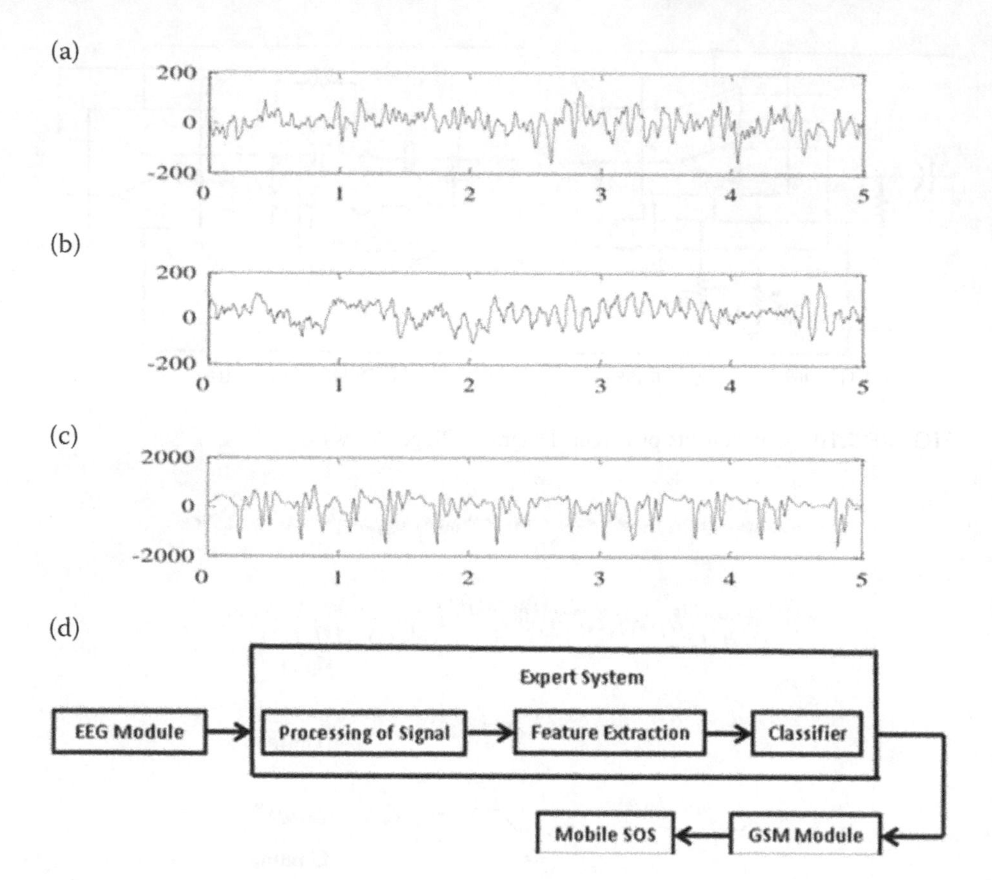

FIGURE 5.12 (a) Normal, (b) Interictal (period between seizues), (c) Ictal (epileptic), (d) Block diagram of nack checker to detect seizure.

3. Resistors
   a. 12 Ω – 2 Pcs
   b. 220 Ω – 1 Pcs
   c. 560 Ω – 1 Pcs
   d. 22 KΩ – 2 Pcs
   e. 47 KΩ – 1 Pcs
   f. 100 KΩ – 2 Pcs
   g. 180 KΩ – 2 Pcs
   h. 220 KΩ – 1 Pcs
   i. 270 KΩ – 2 Pcs
   j. 1 MΩ – 1 Pcs
4. 3.5 mm connector
5. Rechargeable battery
6. Electrode supplies

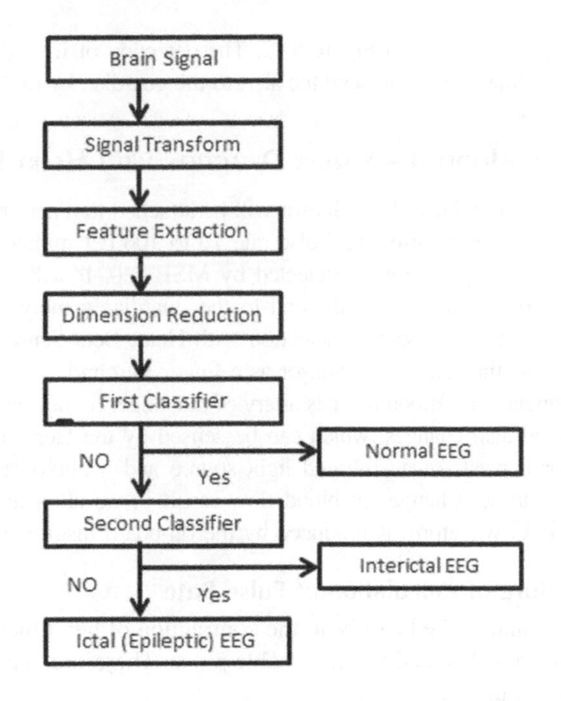

FIGURE 5.13 Flow Diagram of Detecting Epileptic Signal.

In Figure 5.7, a single op-amp is presented by a box after the amplifier. In Figure 5.8(a) an instrumentation amplifier takes two voltages as i/p, and results in the difference between the multiplication of two voltages by some gain. Pin 1 to 8 are used to change the gain by modifying the value of the resistor. In Figure 5.8(b) two 60 Hz "notch" filters are used to reduce interference before applying the gain to circuit and after picking up. In Figure 5.9(c) a 2-pole 7.23 Hz High Pass Filter results in the circuit outputs data that is reduced to about 71% of its original value. The filter consists of two poles. Double-pole design is more advantageous as it reduces data by a factor of about 56 by the time it gets to 1 Hz, while a single pole would only reduce it by a factor of about 7.5. The resistor and capacitor in parallel provide extra filtering of high frequencies on a 31 Hz low-pass filter in In Figures 5.9(d) and 5.10(f) a 60 Hz notch filter is used, finally to reduce the remaining noise.

The circuit in Figure 5.7 can be powered by 2.9 V batteries. For this, two cells are connected on each side of the op-amps with –9 V to 9 V of power. Positive lead of first cell should connect to positive power supply line and the negative lead to the ground. On the other hand, positive lead of first cell should be connecting to the ground and the negative lead to the positive power supply line. The challenge of the circuit is reducing noise at some extent to get a good signal into the computer by obtaining the data.

In Figure 5.13, the EEG module will receive different brain signals having different frequencies. The received signals will be sent to the expert system where the signals will be getting processed for simplifying process. The simplified signal will be identified with the frequency level by feature extraction process. After reducing the dimension of signal, the classifier will classify the signal as Normal EEG, Interictal (period between seizures)

EEG, and Ictal (epileptic) EEG in Figure 5.12. The detection of Ictal signal will be forwarded to GSM module which will send the alert to the guardian by mobile SMS service.

5.3.3 Proposed Model 3 – Seizure Detection with Heart Beat Sensor

In our third approach, one Heart Beat Sensor will be attached to a person as a finger ring whose work is to count the pulse rate. Pulse rate 70 to 100 per minute is considered as normal. Thus, abnormal pulse rate is detected by MSP 430. It will send the signal to GSM module and finally the alert will send to the guardian's mobile. Figure 5.14 illustrates the block diagram of seizure detection with Heart Beat Sensor.

Figure 5.15 shows the Heart Beat Sensor as a finger ring and the place in the finger where to put the finger ring. Blood reaches artery of our finger tip during heart beat. Thus, the volume of blood also changes, which can be sensed by the Heart Beat Sensor. The Heart Beat Sensor consists of an infrared light source and a photodetector to find the change in blood volume. Changes in blood flow result in variation in the photo diode through which a PPG waveform is produced by the on-board instrumentation.

5.3.3.1 Procedure of Calculation of Pulse Rate

The pulse rate is equal to the heart beat; the contraction of heart increases the blood pressure in the arteries that lead to a noticeable pulse. Therefore, a direct measure of heart rate is called pulse rate.

1. Place the tips of index, second, and third fingers on the palm side of another wrist below the base of thumb.
2. Press lightly with fingers until you feel the blood pulsing beneath fingers. Moves fingers slightly up or down until feel the pulsing.
3. Use a watch with a second hand or look at a clock with a second hand.
4. Count the beats feel for 10 seconds. Multiply this number by 6 to get pulse rate per minute.

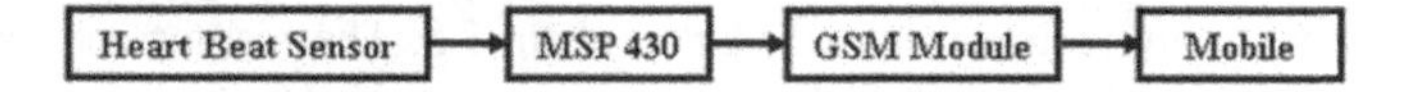

FIGURE 5.14 Block Diagram of Seizure Detection with Heart Beat Sensor.

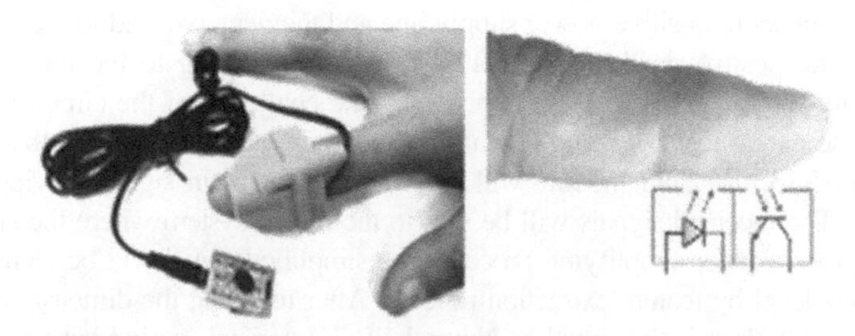

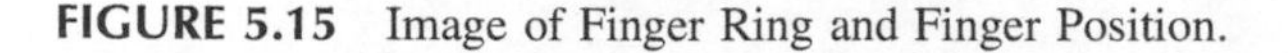

FIGURE 5.15 Image of Finger Ring and Finger Position.

Count pulse = __________beats in 10 seconds × 6
= __________beats per minute

A person having 13 beats in 10 seconds, therefore total count pulse of him/her is 78 beats per minute, i.e., Normal Pulse Rate.

A person having 11 beats in 10 seconds, therefore total count pulse of him/her is 66 beats per minute, i.e., Abnormal Pulse Rate.

5.3.3.2 Normal Pulse Rate

a. Children (age 6–15): 70–100 beats per minute
b. Adult (age 18 and over): 60–100 beats per minute

Figure 5.16 displays the circuit diagram of Heart Beat Sensor [24]. The circuit diagram consists of a light detector and a bright red LED. When a finger is placed in the LED detector, it detects the finger and a large amount of light starts to pass and spread. So, the LED should be of very bright intensity. The finger becomes opaque when heart pumps the blood in the blood vessels. Thus, the detector receives less quantity of light from the LED. The signal of the detector varies with each pulse. Finally, the signal is converted to an electrical pulse. Then, the electrical signal gets amplified and triggered through an amplifier which gives an output of +5 V logic level signal.

Figure 5.17 shows the workflow diagram of detecting seizure using Heart Beat Sensor. The electrical signal gets detected by the Heart Beat Sensor. The signal gets amplified by the amplifier and reaches to MSP430. If MSP430 senses the pulse rate which is normal for a human being then the detection is completed. Otherwise, it

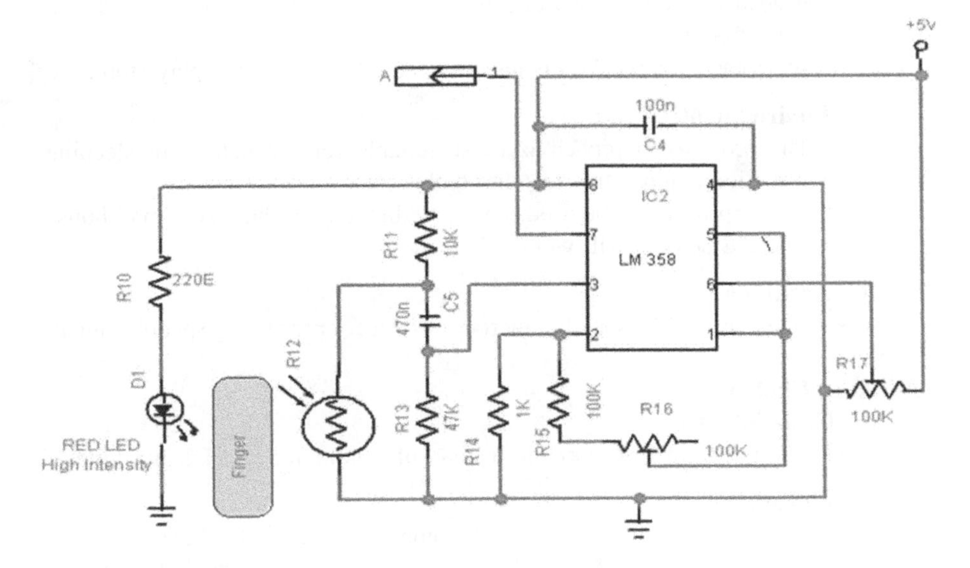

FIGURE 5.16 Circuit Diagram of Heart Beat Sensor.

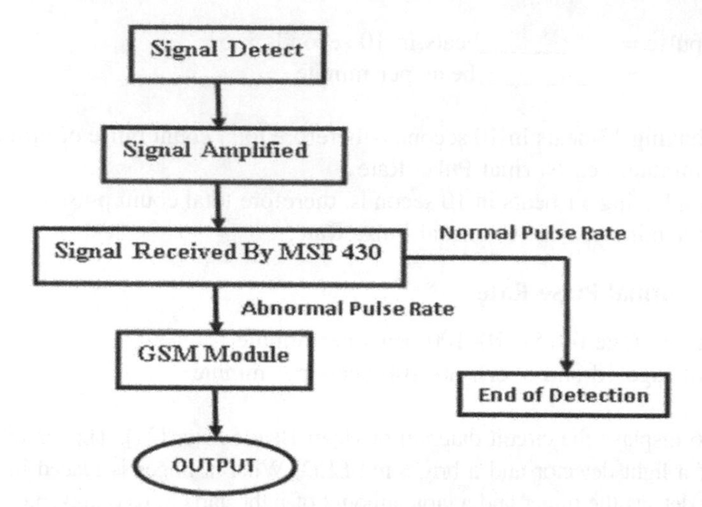

FIGURE 5.17 Workflow Diagram of Finding Seizure Using Heart Beat Sensor.

forwards the sensed abnormal pulse rate to the GSM module. Through which guardian can be alerted of patient's seizer attack and they can take the necessary action.

5.4 DISCUSSION

A. **Close Circuit Seizure Detector**

1. **Cost-Effective**
    - The proposed approach used two smartphones (one may be an old one) instead of CCTV for video feeding and capturing, thus rendering it cost-effective.
    - At Home Monitor App is also available for free in the play store.
2. **Environment**
    - The proposed approach is most suitable for the patient in sleeping condition comparative to other techniques.
    - This approach can be used mostly within a car or home or small house where Bluetooth will work.
3. **Accuracy**
    - Due to use of the specific microcontroller for processing specific signal.

B. **Neck Choker**

1. **Cost-Effective**
    - Due to use of EEG module instead of installation of EEG machine.
2. **Flexibility**
    - A person can wear it without any complexity because total expert system is embedded in the Neck Choker which is also comfortable to wear.

3. **Environment**
    - The proposed system can be used in anytime including sleeping time also.

C. **Seizure detection with Heart Beat Sensor**
1. **Cost-Effective**
2. **Flexibility**
    - Small size as it is used as a finger ring and is also comfortable to wear.
3. **Environment**
    - The proposed system can be used in anytime including sleeping time also.
4. **Accuracy**
    - Due to use of specific microcontroller for processing specific signal.

5.5 CONCLUSION

We proposed three different systems for detecting epilepsy attack as early as possible. The three proposed methods are suitable for various environments and give accurate result in each situation.

Each of the approaches has advantages which have been discussed earlier. According to Epilepsy Society, UK, around 600 people die due to unexpected death due to epilepsy. As per WHO, epilepsy affects nearly 50 million people around the world – 80% live in low- and middle-income countries. An estimated 70% of people with epilepsy could be seizure-free if properly diagnosed and treated. Thus, our three proposed models can be very helpful and efficient in detecting the seizures at early stage which will lead the people to become seizure-free. Some technical knowledge is mandatory for the implementation of any one of the three proposed models on the patients. Access to smartphone is mandatory for using the models for getting the alert for seizure detection of the respective patient.

REFERENCES

1. Mayo Clinic. Epilepsy. (2020). https://www.mayoclinic.org/diseases-conditions/epilepsy/symptoms-causes/syc-20350093
2. Gandhi, V., & Singh, J. (2020). An automated review of body sensor networks research patterns and trends. *Journal of Industrial Information Integration*, *18*, 100132.
3. Negra, R., Jemili, I., & Belghith, A. (2016). Wireless body area networks: Applications and technologies. *Procedia Computer Science*, *83*, 1274–1281.
4. Jovanov, E., & Milenkovic, A. (2011). Body area networks for ubiquitous healthcare applications: Opportunities and challenges. *Journal of Medical Systems*, *35*(5), 1245–1254.
5. Al Masud, S. M. R. (2013). Study and analysis of scientific scopes, issues and challenges towards developing a righteous wireless body area network. *International Journal of Soft Computing and Engineering (IJSCE)*, *3*(2), 243–251.
6. Adibi, S. (Ed.). (2015). *Mobile health: A technology road map* (Vol. 5). Springer.
7. Khosropanah, P., Ramli, A. R., Abbasi, M. R., Marhaban, M. H., & Ahmedov, A.

(2020). A hybrid unsupervised approach toward EEG epileptic spikes detection. *Neural Computing and Applications*, *32*(7), 2521–2532.
8. Yol, S., Ozdemir, M. A., Akan, A., & Chaparro, L. F. (2018, November). Detection of epileptic seizures by the analysis of EEG signals using empirical mode decomposition. In *2018 Medical Technologies National Congress (TIPTEKNO)* (pp. 1–4). IEEE.
9. Petkov, G., Kalitzin, S., Demuru, M., Widman, G., Suffczynski, P., & da Silva, F. H. L. (2018, December). Computational model exploration of stimulation based paradigm for detection of epileptic systems. In *APPIS* (pp. 324–335). IOS Press.
10. Suffczynski, P., da Silva, F. L., Parra, J., Velis, D., & Kalitzin, S. (2005). Epileptic transitions: Model predictions and experimental validation. *Journal of Clinical Neurophysiology*, *22*(5), 288–299.
11. Suffczynski, P., Da Silva, F. H. L., Parra, J., Velis, D. N., Bouwman, B. M., Van Rijn, C. M., … & Kalitzin, S. (2006). Dynamics of epileptic phenomena determined from statistics of ictal transitions. *IEEE Transactions on Biomedical Engineering*, *53*(3), 524–532.
12. Lee, K., Khoo, H. M., Lina, J. M., Dubeau, F., Gotman, J., & Grova, C. (2018). Disruption, emergence and lateralization of brain network hubs in mesial temporal lobe epilepsy. *NeuroImage: Clinical*, *20*, 71–84.
13. Borujeny, G. T., Yazdi, M., Keshavarz-Haddad, A., & Borujeny, A. R. (2013). Detection of epileptic seizure using wireless sensor networks. *Journal of Medical Signals and Sensors*, *3*(2), 63.
14. Panahi, S., Aram, Z., Jafari, S., Ma, J., & Sprott, J. C. (2017). Modeling of epilepsy based on chaotic artificial neural network. *Chaos, Solitons & Fractals*, *105*, 150–156.
15. Gao, Y., Zheng, J., Li, Y., Guo, D., Wang, M., Cui, X., & Ye, W. (2018). Abnormal default-mode network homogeneity in patients with temporal lobe epilepsy. *Medicine*, *97*(26).
16. Tailby, C., Kowalczyk, M. A., & Jackson, G. D. (2018). Cognitive impairment in epilepsy: The role of reduced network flexibility. *Annals of Clinical and Translational Neurology*, *5*(1), 29–40.
17. Klugah-Brown, B., Luo, C., He, H., Jiang, S., Armah, G. K., Wu, Y., … & Yao, D. (2019). Altered dynamic functional network connectivity in frontal lobe epilepsy. *Brain Topography*, *32*(3), 394–404.
18. Li, F., Liang, Y., Zhang, L., Yi, C., Liao, Y., Jiang, Y., … & Xu, P. (2019). Transition of brain networks from an interictal to a preictal state preceding a seizure revealed by scalp EEG network analysis. *Cognitive Neurodynamics*, *13*(2), 175–181.
19. Liu, H., & Zhang, P. (2018). Phase synchronization dynamics of neural network during seizures. *Computational and Mathematical Methods in Medicine*, *2018*.
20. Hebbink, J., Meijer, H., Huiskamp, G., van Gils, S., & Leijten, F. (2017). Phenomenological network models: Lessons for epilepsy surgery. *Epilepsia*, *58*(10), e147–e151.
21. Xie, K., Zhang, S., Dong, S., Li, S., Yu, C., Xu, K., … & Wu, Z. (2017). Portable wireless electrocorticography system with a flexible microelectrodes array for epilepsy treatment. *Scientific Reports*, *7*(1), 1–8.
22. Drenthen, G. S., Backes, W. H., Rouhl, R. P., Vlooswijk, M. C., Majoie, M. H., Hofman, P. A., … & Jansen, J. F. (2018). Structural covariance networks relate to the severity of epilepsy with focal-onset seizures. *NeuroImage: Clinical*, *20*, 861–867.
23. Instructables.com. DIY EEG (and ECG) circuit. (2018). https://www.instructables.com/id/DIY-EEG-and-ECG-Circuit/#step2
24. Elprocus. Heartbeat sensor circuit and working operation with 805. (2013). https://www.elprocus.com/heartbeat-sensor-circuit-daigram-working-with-8051/

6 Prediction of Users' Performance in Surgical Augmented Reality Simulation-Based Training Using Machine Learning Techniques

Hamza Ghandorh
College of Computer Science and Engineering, Taibah University, Medina, Saudi Arabia

CONTENTS

6.1 INTRODUCTION

In the neurosurgical field, performing neurosurgical procedures requires hard skills (e.g., medical knowledge, judgment, dexterity) and soft skills (e.g., collaboration, communication, teamwork). All these skills need to be included in the surgeons' training curricula. Neurosurgical procedures necessitate the deliberate training of neurosurgeons for targeting tasks to build expertise in skills in effective ways as soon as possible (Ericsson 2006).

DOI: 10.1201/9781003198796-6

With rise in medical research the utilization of advanced simulation tools has also increased to not only increase patients' wellbeing and safety but also to be used as educational tools and objective assessment tools. The simulation tools provide a mode of evaluation of a hierarchy of surgical tasks within a neurosurgical procedure based on quantitative metrics with accurate and timely feedback. Besides other advanced technologies, medical researchers have utilized AR technology to mimic deliberate training in the neurosurgical field. For example, Abhari et al. (2015) proposed a mixed AR system to facilitate training for planning common neurosurgical procedures, such as brain tumor resection. de Ribaupierre et al. (2015) proposed a VR/AR module that aims to visualize anatomical geometrical meshes that were designed as an extension of a haptic system developed, referred to as NeuroTouch.

There are many advantages to the use of recent advancements in MLCs in medicine. For example, Deep Learning-based systems can learn from physicians' experiences and empower trainees with nonconventional insights. Direct patient care would be achieved by selecting proper treatment methods and in providing robotic surgeries and examinations. Telemedicine would also be accomplished with indirect patient care for remote areas with the help of wearable devices and sensors (Ogilvie and Eggleton 2017). Moreover, AI would pave the way for physicians to effectively find and understand health information from electronic sources to continue to meet patient needs. In addition, AI holds great potential to not only assist in diagnosis, clinical decision-making, and training but also early prediction and prevention, treatment, and personalized medicine (Reznick et al. 2020).

An advanced surgical training curriculum with objective metrics assessments would produce massive amounts of data by which errors and trends would be detected. The advancement of MLCs would facilitate improved healthcare decision-making to understand these data for the prediction of trainees' performance in different medical fields, including neurosurgery. Therefore, the integration of MLCs and AR technology might revolutionize the healthcare profession on many levels. In this work, we have a hypothesis that MLCs will be able to predict subjects' performance during the use of AR simulation. We propose a study concerning investigating the use of MLCs on user performance from the AR simulation training dataset.

This chapter is organized as following: Section 6.2 states some related concepts to this chapter's scope and current related work. Section 6.3 briefly describes a pilot study to measure 14 novice users for neurosurgical targeting-task simulation and the used simulation tool. Section 6.4 illustrates the results of applying MLCs on users' performance datasets for accuracy between actual and predicted values. Section 6.5 and 6.6 comprise the discussion and conclusion of this chapter, respectively.

6.2 BACKGROUND AND RELATED WORK

This section entails some background about AR simulation and an overview of its use in healthcare. Azuma (1997) described AR technology as a variation between actual and virtual environments in which a user sees both of them, and virtual objects are superimposed upon the real world. In other words, AR would not entirely replace users' reality, but it supplies the user's reality. Any AR system combines real and virtual scenes, exposes users for interaction mode in real-time, and all three-dimensional (3D) objects and scenes are registered. Any AR system entails three components: a 3D scene generator, display or modality device, and tracking and sensing equipment.

Medical AR (MAR) systems have been designed to enhance users' perception of reality through overlaying medical computer-generated information upon patients (Pandya 2004; Armstrong et al. 2016; Luciano et al. 2006; Delorme et al. 2012; Hooten et al. 2014; Kramers et al. 2014). The overlay process facilitates direct interaction and maintaining a perception of the surrounding world and underlying events. The systems provide users (i.e., senior residents and trainees) with a visualization mode that entails a synthesized version of anatomic, metabolic, and functional medical data from different sources (Azuma 1997). The visualization mode will be fused upon a patient's organs from different modalities for a specific patient situation. The visualization mode of data could also be examined in detail, distributed, and discussed with trainees and other peers and research communities. Carmigniani and Furht (2011) indicated that MARs had been used to manage clients' medical history, where a physician wears on a head-mounted display (HMD) equipment and scans an organ or a set of organs to see virtual informatics indicating past injuries or illnesses. Another good use of MAR to combat psychological disorders (e.g., Katsaridaphobia or the fear of cockroaches). MAR could also act as visually impaired assistive technology for path navigation.

There are many advantages of simulation-based training for hospitals and trainees. Hospitals can utilize customized simulators as a supplement and afford to recruit as many trainees as possible. The hospitals, thus, can reduce the usage load on operating rooms (ORs) and the senior surgical team for real procedures. Trainees will be exposed to adequate surgical practice anywhere and anytime. They will also receive autonomous surgical training that involves a variety of surgical techniques, anatomies, and pathologies and offers necessary tools to support different surgical specialties and increase procedures' success rates. More importantly, trainees can have a space for errors without the risk of patients' safety. Meola et al. (2017) surveyed AR systems in neurosurgical procedures in human studies and in vivo applications from 1996 until 2015. The authors reported that AR systems are reliable and versatile tools when performing minimally invasive approaches in a wide range of neurosurgical diseases.

When a particular test or metric measure is conducted for a specific aspect of simulation practices, this is referred to as simulation validation. The process of development of validated simulation tools is challenging due to the complex dynamics of real surgical scenarios that include a variety of actors and interconnected surgical steps. Many efforts investigated the design of simulation tools and their validation for real practice. For example, Van Nortwick et al. (2010) conducted a systematic literature review concerning surgical simulation and establishing validity. The authors reported that there is a lack of well-defined validation methodologies by which they diminish massive challenges for training centers. Schout et al. (2010) conducted a systematic literature review concerning subjective and objective validity studies between 1980 and 2008 in surgical simulators. The authors reported that although there are many studies that proposed definitions for subjective and objective types of validity, there are no general guidelines concerning data interpretation. Barsom et al. (2016) conducted a systematic literature review concerning AR systems for education and training in 2015. The authors reported that a combination of face-, construct-, and concurrent validity studies of AR systems in medical fields was missing.

To the best of our knowledge, there are few works that considered the integration of AI techniques and AR simulators' validation. Mirchi et al. (2020) proposed the use of Virtual Operative Assistant, a versatile tool to train and validate novice neurosurgeons by the use of a haptic neurosurgical simulator referred to as NeuroVR. The authors utilized a linear SVM algorithm to show different expertise levels and identify teachable metrics when trainers performed tasks to the simulated ultrasonic aspirator and bipolar trials. The tool acts as an automated and objective feedback platform for complex neurosurgical tasks by which residency directors would maintain formative educational paradigms. The authors reported that there is a potential with regard to integration of MLCs to assess surgical performance.

6.3 METHODOLOGY

Our goal is to investigate the use of various MLCs on user performance from the AR simulation training dataset. This section sheds light on the used methodology in terms of used tools and conducted a pilot study to achieve our goal.

6.3.1 Apparatus

We conducted a pilot study concerns about measuring quantitively the subjects' performance for targeting tasks. The chosen targeting task is about mimicking a neurosurgical task referred to as the placement of an External Ventricular Drain (EVD) (Virtual Med Student 2021) within a surgical operating referred to as Ventriculostomy (Gorman 2010). The task is about the placement of a plastic probe tool (i.e., catheter) and "aims to choose an appropriate burr hole on the skull and blindly placing a catheter through the burr hole to intersect a lateral ventricle to drain cerebrospinal fluid and relieve intracranial pressure" (de Ribaupierre et al. 2015). The probe tool supposed to be targeting an ellipsoid (i.e., target) through its longest axis. The subjects performed "targeting tasks towards a variety of ellipsoids with a different location, rotation, and size (i.e., ellipsoids widths are 0.10, 0.15, 0.05 mm) and from different distances" (de Ribaupierre et al. 2015).

The tasks were performed on a locally developed AR simulator system (Ghandorh et al. 2017) upon virtual 3D anatomical constructs of the human brain and virtual targets, Unity3D game engine (Unity Manual 2017; Vuforia Library 2020). The system included a flat display screen, an external camera, two trackable fiducial markers, and a local machine.

A user performs an EVD placement task in a virtual scene, including an EVD target, the lateral ventricle. The user is holding a virtual probe tool and navigating into the 3D scene toward the EVD target. The user needs to inject the probe tool into the optimal entry point of the target to achieve accurate penetration (Ghandorh et al. 2017).

The targets are predefined entry points to the lateral ventricle meshes based on a senior neurosurgeon's insights for real scenarios. The smaller the targets are and those with narrow angles, the longer time it takes to target. The combination of

Vuforia API and Unity game engine combination allowed us to generate different prototypes concerning adjustable target specifications.

6.3.2 Pilot Study

This study recruited 14 graduate students intended to serve as trainees. The trainees performed 378 trials[1] (i.e., 14 user × 27 targets) in total, where each subject completed a single task against a single target, and each subject experienced 27 scenarios in random order. An overview of the subjects is depicted in Table 6.1. The subjects came from different backgrounds, gender, and skill levels, where some portion of the subject has used simulation tools, and the other portion has not used simulation tools previously.

6.3.3 Human Evaluation Technique

In terms of the evaluation of novices' performance, surgical competency through the manipulation of physical objects is vital. Surgical tasks involve the manipulation of a physical object or psychomotor task in multiple degrees-of-freedom (DoF) movements. Thus, a 3D extension of Fitts' law (Murata and Iwase 2001; MacKenzie 1992) might be used to assess novices' performance. Fitts (1954) investigated performance in human psychomotor behavior (e.g., moving an object from one area to another area) through various single DoF movement tasks. Fitts' Law states that "the meantime to perform a movement and selection task is logarithmically related to the target's width and the distance to the target." In other

TABLE 6.1
Subjects Demographics

Subject ID	Age	Gender	Medical background	Simulation background
User01	20–29	Female	Yes	Yes
User02	20–29	Male	Yes	Yes
User03	20–29	Female	No	Yes
User04	20–29	Male	No	Yes
User05	30–39	Female	No	Yes
User06	20–29	Male	No	Yes
User07	30–39	Male	No	Yes
User08	20–29	Male	No	No
User09	40–49	Male	No	No
User10	30–39	Male	No	No
User11	40–49	Male	No	No
User12	40–49	Male	No	No
User13	20–29	Male	No	No
User14	20–29	Male	No	No

words, every user, the more precise he/she makes a specific movement slower he/she will move. Fitts' law concerns to determine human performance as a trade-off between accuracy and speed through Index of Performance (IP) (bit/second) metric, which is measured as Equation 6.1:

$$IP = \frac{\log_2\left(\frac{A}{W} + 1\right)}{MT} = \frac{ID}{MT} \quad (6.1)$$

Where *IP* represents the required time needed to accomplish a task, Index of Difficulty (*ID*) is how accurate and fast the participants were to complete the tasks. *A* is the distance between the starting point of the user and the center of the targets (mm). *W* is a target width. Table 6.2 shows a sample of targeting tasks description (i.e., dataset features) for 14 participants.

6.3.4 Machine Learning Classifiers (MLCs)

To achieve our goal, we tried various MLCs: K-Nearest Neighbors (k-NN), Nearest Centroid (NC), Support Vector Machine (SVM), and Decision Trees (DT). NC is an extremely fast classifier that is introduced by Lilien et al. (2003). From extracting mass spectra feature using Principle Components Analysis (PCA) and Linear Discriminant Analysis (LDA).

DT (Theobald 2017; Magee 1964) is a classification technique that entails recursively dividing input data samples into branches to construct a tree-like structure. It consists of one root node where the tree starts, the number of internal nodes, and the leaf node is the final node. Each node holds a class label attached to it. Any node representing the leaf node or continues to split depends on several attributes by which a decision can be made. Kolomogorov Complexity, entropy, relative entropy, etc., are commonly used to select attributes (Leonard 2017).

NC uses a similar approach as used by k-NN (Soucy and Mineau 2001), but instead of using K nearest training samples, it uses the nearest mean approach for classification. In this classifier, the whole vector space is divided into regions which are centered on centroid, one for each of the class. The instance that has the nearest distance with the centroid is classified with that particular class (Wang and Zhao 2012).

SVM had been used for regression and classification tasks. It aims to locate a hyperplane in multiple features to unique organize a portion of data points in a particular space. A hyperplane is decision boundaries to help classify the data points (Nayak et al. 2015).

6.3.5 Performance Measures

We used two evaluation criteria to compare the accuracy between subjects' performance values resulted from Fitts' Law and the two MLCs. As reported through the literature, Mean Magnitude of Relative Error (MMRE) and average PRED(A) are used (Malhotra and Jain 2011), which are listed in Equations 6.2 and 6.3, respectively:

TABLE 6.2
Sample of Targeting Tasks Description Within the AR-Based Neurosurgical Simulator

Target width (W) (mm)	Amplitude (A) (cm)	Index of Difficulty (ID) (bit)	Movement time (MT) (second)	Index of Performance (IP) (bit/second)
0.1	280.53	11.45	13	0.88
0.05	124.99	11.29	2	5.64
0.15	89.46	9.22	6	1.54
0.15	11.98	6.34	1	6.34
0.05	536.4	13.39	8	1.67
0.05	44.24	9.79	7	1.4
0.15	1,088.55	12.83	7	1.83
0.05	192.63	11.91	1	11.91
0.1	90.85	9.83	6	1.64
0.15	95.96	9.32	24	0.39
0.1	110.49	10.11	16	0.63
0.1	43.04	8.75	25	0.35
0.05	919.73	14.17	108	0.13
0.1	4.69	5.58	1	5.58
0.1	257.75	11.33	11	1.03
0.05	787.74	13.94	25	0.56
0.1	1.8	4.25	1	4.25
0.05	11.7	7.88	2	3.94
0.15	175.89	10.2	6	1.7
0.1	373.55	11.87	17	0.7
0.15	91.01	9.25	15	0.62
0.15	1185	12.95	35	0.37
0.1	231.69	11.18	4	2.79
0.15	476.15	11.63	12	0.97
0.05	313.49	12.61	10	1.26
0.1	275.22	11.43	17	0.67
0.15	1,202.59	12.97	28	0.46
0.05	81.15	10.67	37	0.29
0.05	55.81	10.13	5	2.03
0.15	693.32	12.17	11	1.11
0.1	493.07	12.27	55	0.22
0.15	945.41	12.62	14	0.9
0.05	258.58	12.34	61	0.2
0.15	375.44	11.29	55	0.21
0.15	3.12	4.45	10	0.44
0.15	333.23	11.12	1	11.12
0.05	626.48	13.61	6	2.27

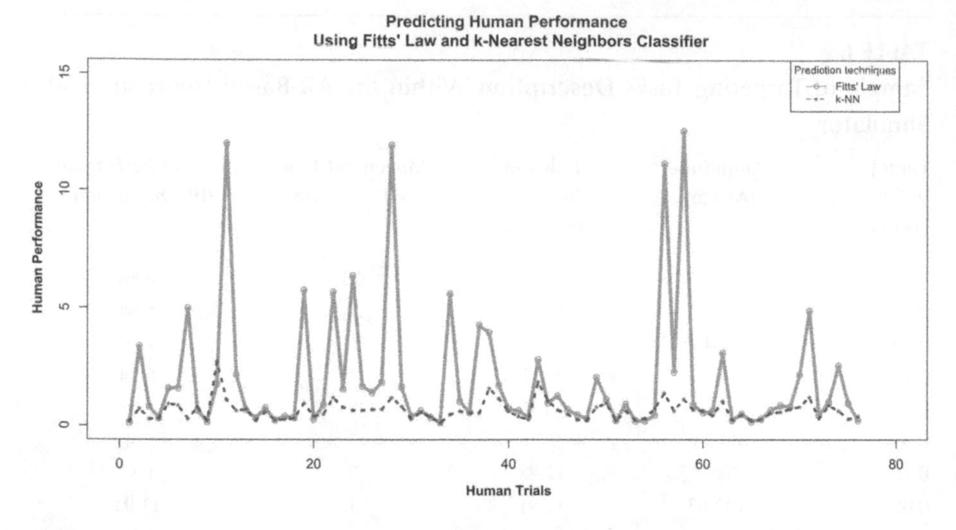

FIGURE 6.1 Actual and Predicted Performance Using Fitts' Law and k-NN Classifier.

$$MMRE = \frac{1}{n} \sum_{i=1}^{n} \frac{|P_i - A_i|}{|A_i|} \tag{6.2}$$

$\boldsymbol{P_i}$ is the predicted value for datapoint i. $\boldsymbol{A_i}$ is the actual value for datapoint i. $\boldsymbol{n}$ is the total number of data points.

$$PRED(A) = \frac{d}{n} \tag{6.3}$$

$\boldsymbol{d}$ is the value of $\boldsymbol{MRE}$ where data points have less than or equal to $\boldsymbol{A}$.

6.4 FINDINGS

The dataset features W, A, ID, and MT were used as input to both MLCs, and the value of *IP* is predicted by both. k-NN, NC, SVM gave the prediction results, and DT, shown in Figures 6.1 to 6.4, respectively.

Figure 6.5 depicts mean magnitude relative error for the used MLCs.

Comparing values for minimum MMRE and Maximum PRED(A), DT showed better performance than NC, k-NN, and SVM, which is shown in Tables 6.3 to 6.6, respectively.

6.5 DISCUSSION

As medical big data have been investigated to analyze medical operation indicators and provide data support for medical decision-making, they could be utilized to build better predictive models and drive autonomous healthcare assessment models. These predictive models will facilitate the offering of high-quality healthcare practice and more understanding (Elezabeth et al. 2018; Hassanien et al. 2019).

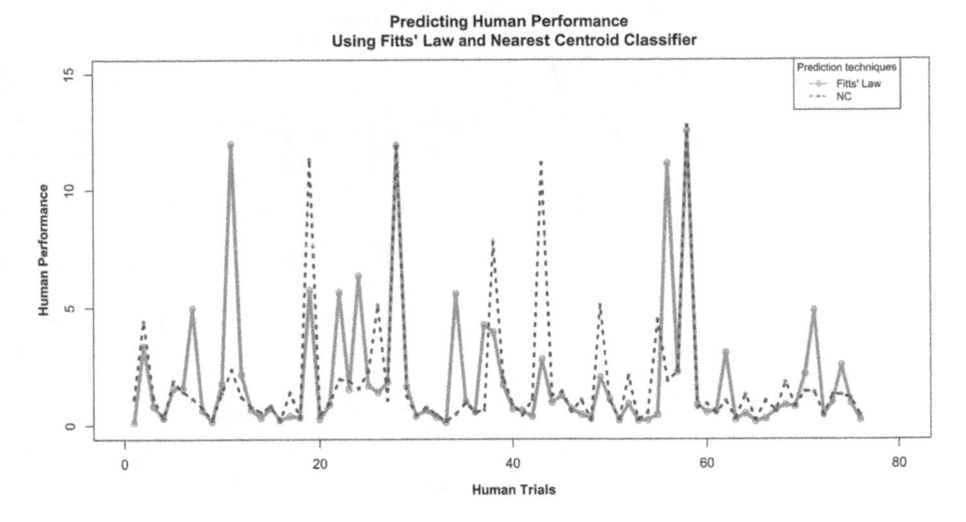

FIGURE 6.2 Actual and Predicted Performance Using Fitts' Law and NC Classifier.

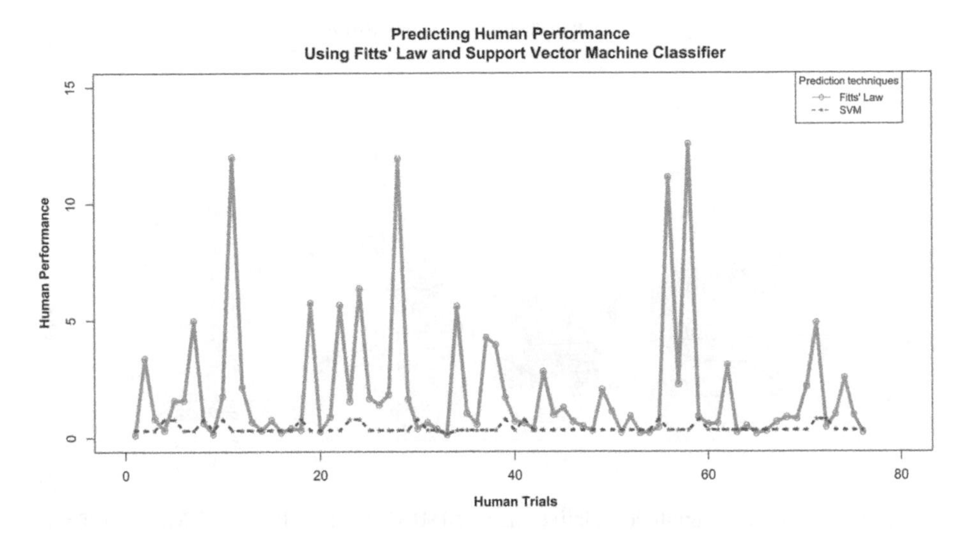

FIGURE 6.3 Actual and Predicted Performance Using Fitts' Law and SVM Classifier.

The dataset entails 378 data points. From these 378 data points, 80% (302) was used for MLCs training, and the remaining 20% (76) was used for MLCs validation.

In this work, we compared various MLCs on the AR simulation tool and user performance dataset. The dataset entails a variety of details about activity-related attributes, and we only used five features. The dataset included other features related to ground truth features about the subjects (e.g., simulation background, the position towards the target, used hand). Task-related attributes (e.g., timestamp, event type, probe tool transformations), 3D construct transformations (translation,

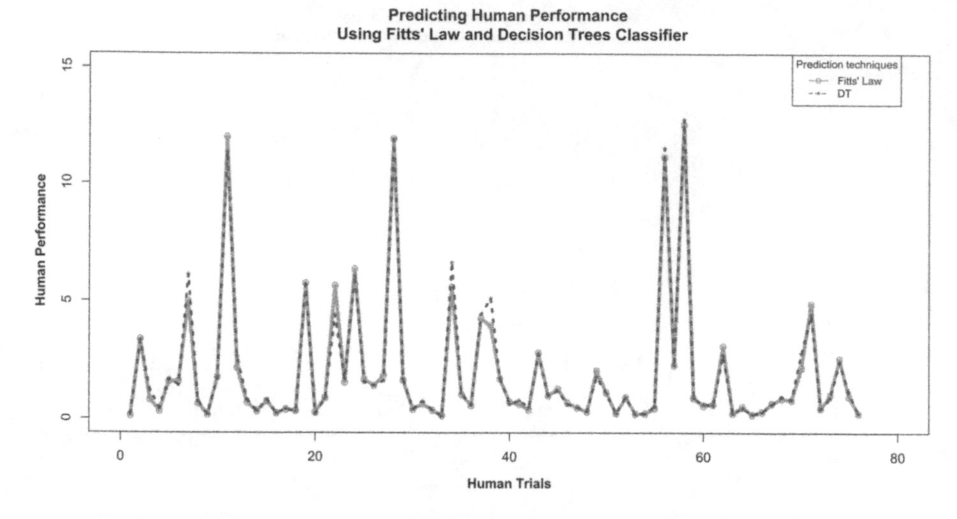

FIGURE 6.4 Actual and Predicted Performance Using Fitts' Law and DT Classifier.

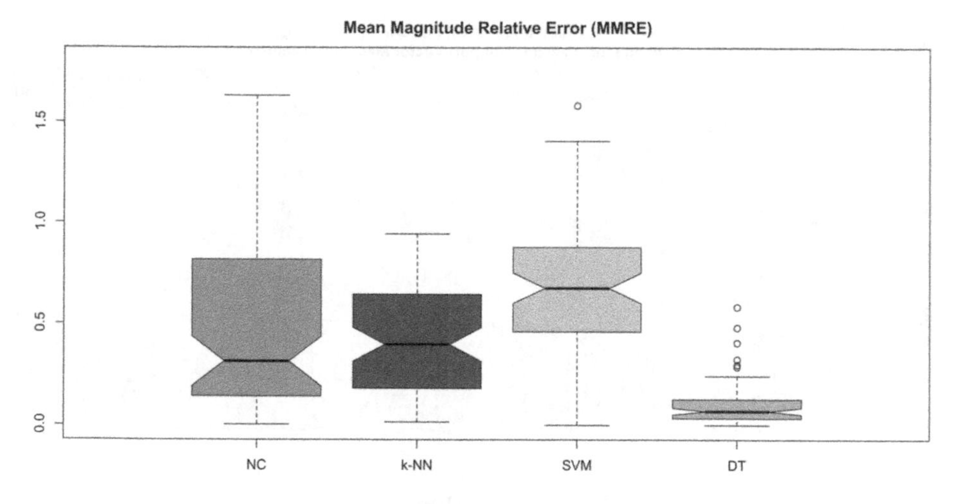

FIGURE 6.5 Mean Magnitude Relative Error (MMRE) for NC, k-NN, SVM, and DT.

TABLE 6.3
MMRE and Maximum PRED(A) from NC Classifier

MMRE	PRED (25)	PRED (50)	PRED (75)
0.79148	0.447368	0.631579	0.710526

TABLE 6.4
MMRE and Maximum PRED(A) from k-NN Classifier

MMRE	PRED (25)	PRED (50)	PRED (75)
0.430	0.329	0.618	0.816

TABLE 6.5
MMRE and Maximum PRED(A) from SVM Classifier

MMRE	PRED (25)	PRED (50)	PRED (75)
0.655	0.145	0.289	0.579

TABLE 6.6
MMRE and Maximum PRED(A) from DT Classifier

MMRE	PRED (25)	PRED (50)	PRED (75)
0.105392	0.828947	0.921053	0.947368

rotation, scaling), other virtual objects in the virtual scene were included in the dataset. Event-related attributes (e.g., probe-to-target distance, incidence angle, elapsed time) also were included in the dataset. Each trial showed how each subject performed the task in terms of activity-related attributes, where the tasks might be emulated under the same circumstances for further analysis.

6.6 CONCLUSION AND FUTURE WORK

Maintaining high-quality and reasonable healthcare services is challenging for all individuals. Thus, innovative approaches become necessary for rapid complexity of healthcare and the handling of growing data. This work aimed to explore the possibility of prediction of subjects' performance based on the comparison of Nearest Centroid and Decision Trees classifier and traditional human performance assessment methodology (Fitts' Law) within a 3D environment. The subjects' performed 3D targeting tasks through a pilot study with 376 trials to demonstrate their learning curve and calculate their performance objectively and quantitively. The results depicted that DT had a low mean error for predicting user performance with an MMRE value of 0.105. We suggest that DT is proper to predict user performance in the used AR simulation dataset.

Big data would be generated from advanced AR simulation tools and their use in surgical training and assessment. AR and MLCs will act as critical players for efficient and more versatile healthcare as a practice and as an education. MLCs will serve as a vital stimulus for modernizing healthcare applications. For instance, data-driven run-time recommendation systems in ORs with AR visualization mode, AR simulation tools with playback capabilities would be a reality in the foreseeable future. MLCs could detect trends from generated AR datasets from previously performed surgeries, and they ought to recommend a specific action in a particular situation with benefits and risks. They have the potential to demonstrate how a well-known neurosurgeon in a particular time or place solved an issue as a part of telemedicine practice. MLCs could serve as autonomous mentors or evaluators for joiner surgeons for entry, intermediate, and advance surgery scenarios.

Various Deep Learning classifiers would help expand our understanding of human performance in AR environments. Artificial Neural Network (ANN) or Long-term Short Memory (LSTM) classifiers would be the next stage in our investigation to examine whether performance prediction would be improved.

NOTE

1 Trial is a case when a user performs an individual targeting task towards an AR-based neurosurgical simulator target in the 3D scene.

REFERENCES

Abhari, Kamyar, John S. H. Baxter, Elvis C. S. Chen, Ali R. Khan, Terry M. Peters, Sandrine de Ribaupierre, and Roy Eagleson. "Training for Planning Tumour Resection: Augmented Reality and Human Factors." *IEEE Transactions on Biomedical Engineering* 62, no. 6 (June 2015): 1466–1477. 10.1109/TBME.2014.2385874.

Armstrong, Ryan, Trinette Wright, Sandrine de Ribaupierre, and Roy Eagleson. "Augmented Reality for Neurosurgical Guidance: An Objective Comparison of Planning Interface Modalities." In *Medical Imaging and Augmented Reality*, edited byGuoyan Zheng, Hongen Liao, Pierre Jannin, Philippe Cattin, and Su-Lin Lee, 9805: 233–243. Cham: Springer International Publishing, 2016. 10.1007/978-3-319-43775-0_21.

Azuma, Ronald T. "A Survey of Augmented Reality." *Presence: Teleoperators and Virtual Environments* 6, no. 4 (August 1997): 355–385. 10.1162/pres.1997.6.4.355.

Barsom, E. Z., M. Graafland, and M. P. Schijven. "Systematic Review on the Effectiveness of Augmented Reality Applications in Medical Training." *Surgical Endoscopy* 30, no. 10 (October 2016): 4174–4183. 10.1007/s00464-016-4800-6.

Carmigniani, Julie, and Borko Furht. "Augmented Reality: An Overview." In *Handbook of Augmented Reality*, edited byBorko Furht, 3–46. New York, NY: Springer New York, 2011. 10.1007/978-1-4614-0064-6_1.

de Ribaupierre, Sandrine, Ryan Armstrong, Dayna Noltie, Matt Kramers, and Roy Eagleson. "VR and AR Simulator for Neurosurgical Training." In *2015 IEEE Virtual Reality (VR)*, 147–148. Arles, Camargue, Provence, France: IEEE, 2015. 10.1109/VR.2015.7223338.

Delorme, Sébastien, Denis Laroche, Robert DiRaddo, and Rolando F. Del Maestro. "NeuroTouch." *Operative Neurosurgery* 71, no. suppl_1 (September 1, 2012): ons32–ons42. 10.1227/NEU.0b013e318249c744.

Elezabeth, Laura et al. "The Role of Big Data Mining in Healthcare Applications." *2018 7th International Conference on Reliability, Infocom Technologies and Optimization (Trends and Future Directions) (ICRITO)*, IEEE, 2018: 256-260, Noida, India

Ericsson, K. Anders. "The Influence of Experience and Deliberate Practice on the Development of Superior Expert Performance." In *The Cambridge Handbook of Expertise and Expert Performance*, edited byK. Anders Ericsson, Neil Charness, Paul J. Feltovich, and Robert R. Hoffman, 683–704. Cambridge: Cambridge University Press, 2006. 10.1017/CBO9780511816796.038.

Fitts, Paul M. "The Information Capacity of the Human Motor System in Controlling the Amplitude of Movement." *Journal of Experimental Psychology* 47, no. 6 (1954): 381–391. 10.1037/h0055392.

Ghandorh, Hamza, Justin Mackenzie, Roy Eagleson, and Sandrine de Ribaupierre. "Development of Augmented Reality Training Simulator Systems for Neurosurgery Using Model-Driven Software Engineering." In *2017 IEEE 30th Canadian Conference on Electrical and Computer Engineering (CCECE)*, 1–6. Windsor, ON: IEEE, 2017. 10.1109/CCECE.2017.7946843.

Gorman Peter B. "Fundamentals of Operative Techniques in Neurosurgery." edited by E. Sander Connolly, G. M. McKhannII, J. Huang, T. F. Choudhri, R. J. Komotar, Second Edition. Thieme Medical Publishers, Inc, 2010.

Hassanien, Aboul Ella, Nilanjan Dey, and Surekha Borra, eds. *Medical Big Data and Internet of Medical Things: Advances, Challenges and Applications*. Boca Raton: CRC Press/ Taylor & Francis Group, 2019.

Hooten, Kristopher G., J. Richard Lister, Gwen Lombard, David E. Lizdas, Samsun Lampotang, Didier A. Rajon, Frank Bova, and Gregory J.A. Murad. "Mixed Reality Ventriculostomy Simulation: Experience in Neurosurgical Residency." *Operative Neurosurgery* 10, no. 4 (December 1, 2014): 565–576. 10.1227/NEU.0000000000000503.

Kramers, Matthew, Ryan Armstrong, Saeed M. Bakhshmand, Aaron Fenster, Sandrine de Ribaupierre, and Roy Eagleson. "Evaluation of a Mobile Augmented Reality Application for Image Guidance of Neurosurgical Interventions." *Studies in Health Technology and Informatics* 196 (2014): 204–208.

Leonard, LC. "Web-based behavioral modeling for continuous user authentication (CUA)." Advances in Computers 105, (2017): 1–44, doi:10.1016/bs.adcom.2016.12.001.

Lilien, Ryan H, Hany Farid, and Bruce R.Donald. "Probabilistic Disease Classification of Expression-Dependent Proteomic Data from Mass Spectrometry of Human Serum." *Journal of Computational Biology* 10, no. 6 (December 2003): 925–946. 10.1089/1 06652703322756159.

Luciano, Cristian, Pat Banerjee, G. Michael Lemole, and Fady Charbel. "Second Generation Haptic Ventriculostomy Simulator Using the ImmersiveTouch System." *Studies in Health Technology and Informatics* 119 (2006): 343–348.

MacKenzie, I. Scott. "Fitts' Law as a Research and Design Tool in Human-Computer Interaction." *Human–Computer Interaction* 7, no. 1 (March 1992): 91–139. 10.1207/ s15327051hci0701_3.

Magee, John. "Decision Trees for Decision Making." Harvard Business Review, July 1, 1964. https://hbr.org/1964/07/decision-trees-for-decision-making.

Malhotra, Ruchika, and Ankita Jain. "Software Effort Prediction Using Statistical and Machine Learning Methods." *International Journal of Advanced Computer Science and Applications* 2, no. 1 (2011). 10.14569/IJACSA.2011.020122.

Meola, Antonio, Fabrizio Cutolo, Marina Carbone, Federico Cagnazzo, Mauro Ferrari, and Vincenzo Ferrari. "Augmented Reality in Neurosurgery: A Systematic Review." *Neurosurgical Review* 40, no. 4 (October 2017): 537–548. 10.1007/s10143-016-0732-9.

Mirchi, Nykan, Vincent Bissonnette, Recai Yilmaz, Nicole Ledwos, Alexander Winkler-Schwartz, and Rolando F. Del Maestro. "The Virtual Operative Assistant: An Explainable Artificial Intelligence Tool for Simulation-Based Training in Surgery and Medicine." Edited byPaweł Pławiak. *PLOS ONE* 15, no. 2 (February 27, 2020): e0229596. 10.1371/journal.pone.0229596.

Murata, Atsuo, and Hirokazu Iwase. "Extending Fitts' Law to a Three-Dimensional Pointing Task." *Human Movement Science* 20, no. 6 (December 2001): 791–805. 10.1016/S0167-9457(01)00058-6.

Nayak, Janmenjoy, Bighnaraj Naik, and H. S. Behera. "A Comprehensive Survey on Support Vector Machine in Data Mining Tasks: Applications & Challenges." *International Journal of Database Theory and Application* 8, no. 1 (February 28, 2015): 169–186. 10.14257/ijdta.2015.8.1.18.

Ogilvie, Kelvin Kenneth, and Art Eggleton. "Canadian Healthcare System Must Brace for a Technological Revolution." Senate of Canada, October 31, 2017. https://sencanada.ca/en/newsroom/soci-challenge-ahead/.

Pandya, Abhilash. "Medical Augmented Reality System for Image-Guided and Robotic Surgery: Development and Surgeon Factors Analysis - ProQuest." Wayne State University, 2004. https://search.proquest.com/openview/2b3509f6e1a4cfbfc7088c0b35d65208/1?pq-origsite=gscholar&cbl=18750&diss=y.

Reznick, Richard, Ken Harris, Tanya Horsley, and Mohsen Sheikh Hassani. "Task Force Report on Artificial Intelligence and Emerging Digital Technologies." Royal College of Physicians and Surgeons of Canada, February 2020. https://www.royalcollege.ca/rcsite/health-policy/initiatives/ai-task-force-e.

Schout, B. M. A., A. J. M. Hendrikx, F. Scheele, B. L. H. Bemelmans, and A. J. J. A. Scherpbier. "Validation and Implementation of Surgical Simulators: A Critical Review of Present, Past, and Future *Surgical Endoscopy*24, no. 3 (March 2010): 536–546. 10.1007/s00464-009-0634-9.

Soucy, P., and G. W. Mineau. "A Simple KNN Algorithm for Text Categorization." In *Proceedings 2001 IEEE International Conference on Data Mining*, 647–648. San Jose, CA, USA: IEEE Computer Society, 2001. 10.1109/ICDM.2001.989592.

Theobald, Oliver. *Machine Learning for Absolute Beginners: A Plain English Introduction*. 2nd edition. Scatterplot Press, 2017.

Unity Manual. "Unity User Manual (5.5)." Unity Technologies, 2017. https://docs.unity3d.com/550/Documentation/Manual/index.html.

Van Nortwick, Sara S., Thomas S. Lendvay, Aaron R. Jensen, Andrew S. Wright, Karen D. Horvath, and Sara Kim. "Methodologies for Establishing Validity in Surgical Simulation Studies." *Surgery* 147, no. 5 (May 2010): 622–630. 10.1016/j.surg.2009.10.068.

Virtual Med Student. "VirtualMedStudent.Com || How to Place an External Ventricular Drain." Virtual Med Student, March 9, 2021. http://www.virtualmedstudent.com/links/how_to/how_to_place_external_ventricular_drain.html.

Vuforia Library. "Vuforia Developer Portal." PTC Inc., 2020. https://developer.vuforia.com/.

Wang, L., and X. Zhao. "Improved KNN Classification Algorithms Research in Text Categorization." In , –, IEEE (2012). 2nd International Conference on Consumer Electronics, Communications and Networks (CECNet) 1848 1852 10.1109/CECNet.2012.6201850

7 An Ensemble Approach for Argument Mining on Medical Reviews

Abhiruchi Bhattacharya, Kasturi Kumbhar, Padmaja Borwankar, Ariscia Mendes, and Sujata Khedkar

CONTENTS

7.1 INTRODUCTION

There is a huge amount of ongoing research and discovery in the medical domain. Hence, newer improved drugs are coming into the market on a regular basis. These medicines, although effective, may have side effects that may not be discovered during clinical trials. An adverse drug reaction (ADR) is an unwanted or dangerous reaction experienced following the administration of a drug or a combination of drugs. Thus, it becomes necessary not only to see how these drugs react outside of lab tests but also monitor effectiveness.

Online medical drug reviews are a primary source of information about drug effectiveness and adverse reactions, especially in today's highly social networking

DOI: 10.1201/9781003198796-7

driven environment. Patients can freely voice their opinions regarding various medicines through online forums and websites. Loads of such data are available on the Internet, the best part being it comes straight from the users. To learn and understand more about the effects these drugs have on the human body, it is essential to extract meaningful parts and insights from this discourse.

7.1.1 Medical Reviews

Healthcare information and medical big data includes various resources such as scientific literature, medical reports and statistics, electronic health records, curated datasets, and user testimonies in the form of forum discussions, informal reviews, etc. [1]. While medical reports and datasets come with the concerns of maintaining privacy of the individuals alongside authenticity of the data, user reviews are a more informal source of information where users describe their personal experience with a medical treatment or drug. These reviews are helpful for other consumers as well as healthcare analysts and professionals. Consumers can look up to other peoples' accounts and experiences with drug treatments in order to understand the risks and potential side effects of a drug, differentiate between generic and branded versions, and make an informed decision about their healthcare investment. Professionals, on the other hand, can look to user reviews as a primary source of information to find out the behavior of specific drugs in circulation and track their effectiveness and interactions. This becomes significant especially in scenarios related to exploring alternative prescriptions for a new or developing disease, or testing out the behavior of a new treatment. Sentiment analysis classifies text as positive, negative, or neutral that is based on polarity. For example, in emotion-based sentiment classification, text is categorized into emotional states such as happy, sad, angry, etc. The problem here is mainly that only classification is done, there is no exploration as to why the opinion is so. Basically, the reasoning behind it is unknown.

The main issue with consulting user reviews is bulk. User reviews are available in plenty on a multitude of popular websites such as WebMD, drugs.com, and even on social media such as Twitter. Going through these reviews manually becomes infeasible. An information extraction system can highly expedite the process and present significant insights to analysts from high volume data.

7.1.2 Challenges in Handling Medical Reviews

Due to their very nature, user reviews are subjective. Hence, they cannot be completely relied upon as factually true, and so any system that extracts insights from them will at best be a decision support system and cannot replace healthcare professionals completely.

Another challenge associated with text processing on user reviews is that a medical review may use medical terminology in conjunction with natural language, as well as informal terminology, acronyms, punctuations, etc. User reviews also tend to have longer, run-on sentences that express contradictory ideas. Such sentences may need to be segmented into smaller chunks, and irrelevant information needs to be discarded to present the core opinion of the reviewer.

To illustrate, consider the following sentences:

- "I'm also maxed on my Keppra so this is 2 supplement the additional help needed 2 control seizures after a brain cancer surgery"
- "works fast and was effective for me, but the side effects left me in never-never land."

The above two sentences are taken from separate reviews for the drug phenytoin. We can see that both sentences use informal terminology. The first sentence additionally mixes medical terms ("Keppra," "seizures," etc.) with natural language and slang (using "2" instead of "to"). The second sentence presents two attacking ideas: that the medicine was effective, and that the side-effects were significant. Hence, the second sentence can be represented as two clauses, representing one idea each, with an attacking relation between them.

7.2 MOTIVATION

A large amount of data is generated on online platforms with respect to drugs and their effects. Summarization is necessary to provide an overview of this data. Popularly used NLP techniques limit their analysis to shorter words and phrases, in order to obtain intent or sentiment from a given body of text. Argument mining, on the other hand, focuses on analyzing and understanding argument structure from textual data, and consequently can help in gaining a deeper insight into the claims and opinions of the author, and the evidence and rationale behind them.

Automated extraction of relevant arguments and presenting concise information from data can aid decision-making for medical professionals. A decision support system using argument mining can yield a systematic, structured summary of a large volume of drug reviews, which can help medical professionals identify common patterns of reasoning as well as adverse drug reactions.

7.3 RELATED WORK

Argument mining is concerned with analysis of natural language text on a discourse level, i.e., on a deeper level than syntax or semantic analysis. The main goal of artificial argumentation is to be able to model the flow of logic during discourse, or to recognize or formulate logical arguments. Argument mining techniques, hence, find frequent applications on dialectical or opinionated text such as debate transcripts, persuasive essays, forum discussions, etc.

An early exploration of argument representation for artificial argumentation is presented in [2]. It explores many foundational issues of artificial argumentation such as dividing argumentative text into subcomponents (premises, claims, etc.), representing arguments within unstructured text as a relational database and constructing new arguments from this database. Many of these concepts are realized in subsequent research [3,4] using various techniques.

Argument representation can be done in many ways, varying from broad and simplistic to specific and complex. [5] explores a detailed annotation scheme for argument identification from unstructured text using adpositional trees. It uses the Periodic Table of Arguments [6] which gives a detailed breakdown of many types of arguments used in natural language. Generally, arguments are identified or represented as units of text (propositions, claims, premises, etc.) linked with others in dialectical relationships such as entailment, support, attack, etc.

The task of data preprocessing is essential whether the data is structured or unstructured. [7] focuses on the process of EMR (Electronic Medical Records) processing, analyzes the key techniques, and makes an in-depth study on the applications which are developed related to text mining. [8] provides a detailed survey on representation of argumentative texts. It discusses the relationship between the representing argument structure and the rhetorical structure of texts. It provides suggestions for major challenges that are to be addressed in the field of argument mining.

Notable applications of argumentation using artificial intelligence include IBM's Project Debater [9–17] and ArgumenText [18] from Technical University of Darmstadt.

Project Debater is an ongoing project meant to simulate an AI-based debate opponent that can provide claims and premises for or against a given debate topic dynamically. Research areas involved in this project include argument mining, claim stance identification, listening comprehension, as well as argument quality. Initial research related to Project Debater involved creating a framework to fetch arguments related to a particular topic. Levy et al. [14] and Rinott et al. [10] explore supervised learning methods based on logistic regression classifiers to extract context dependent claims and evidence related to a given topic. They use a benchmark dataset of Wikipedia articles, presented in Aharoni et al. [11]. References [12] and [13] expand automatic claim extraction and explore its application towards unsupervised claim detection. [12] considers a syntax wherein the main concept of a sentence is assumed to occur after the word "that." Word2Vec [14] embeddings are used to detect the presence of a main concept and the claim within the sentence is assumed to directly follow the word "that." [13] attempts to improve the coverage of [12] by considering two Bi-LSTM neural networks, one trained on sentences with the aforementioned syntax and the other on a more relaxed structure. While considering a specific syntax might be beneficial in recognizing arguments, the coverage of such methods may not be ideal as a claim or premise can be presented in many ways that may not necessarily align with a single syntax.

ArgumenText [18] is essentially a search engine for argumentative content based on a specific, user-defined topic. One of the initial papers that led to the development of ArgumenText is by Stab and Gurevych [3], which presents several feature sets for machine learning-based argument identification and relation extraction from persuasive essays. For argument identification, each clause within the manually annotated corpus is classified as claim, major claim, premise, or neither. For relationship extraction, pairs of clauses are classified as "support" or "non-support" based on whether the clauses support each other or not. They report structural and lexical features to be the most effective feature sets, and obtain best accuracy using SVM. Aker et al. [19] rigorously tests the feature sets described in [3] along with word embeddings on the original corpus used in [3] as well as the Wikipedia corpus described in [11]. They report that structural and lexical features are the most effective at identification and classification tasks.

Three alternative machine learning approaches towards argument mining are discussed by Lawrence and Reed [20]. First, discourse indicators are considered as a means to identify a connection between arguments, then argument schemes and topic similarity are used to connect those propositions that remain unconnected after the initial step. They report that discourse indicators are effective in recognizing argumentative content, which makes sense intuitively as well. However, discourse indicators give a high-precision, low-recall scenario as not all argumentative content necessarily uses discourse indicators.

Deep learning techniques are often used in argument mining, especially with the development of LSTM [21] (long-short term memory)-based networks that retain information over longer pieces of text and mitigate the vanishing gradient problem. Cocarascu and Toni [4] present a deep learning approach for the extraction of bipolar argumentation frameworks (BAFs) from text, and apply it towards detecting deceptive hotel and restaurant reviews. BAFs are a graph structure that represent the supportive, attacking, or neutral relation as a directed edge between two sentences, or nodes. The initial GloVe [22] embeddings of each pair of sentences in reviews are first given to two parallel neural networks, and the vector representations obtained are summed or concatenated before giving to a softmax classifier for the final classification. Such a graph structure has benefits in that it is highly convenient to visualize the flow of opinion and how it changes between sentences. BAF graphs can also be used to calculate additional scores such as the dialectical strength of a review, which can further be used to filter out spam or contradictory reviews.

Medical reviews are a rich field of study due to the use of medical terminology that can be formed into a lexicon, but user reviews can be challenging because of informal language structure, misspellings, etc. [23] gives a rule-based approach towards argument extraction. They use reviews from two medical websites, Drugs.com and Webmd.com, and employ rule-based classification method to extract arguments from medical drug reviews. Rules were formalized using First Order Logic. Along with user reviews, user ratings for a particular review are also considered for better argument evaluation. The disadvantage of rule-based classification is similar to that seen in [8–11], i.e., coverage might be low and arguments that do not conform to the rules may be lost.

Learning-based methods on the other hand, are much more flexible. [24] adds task-specific information to pretrained word embeddings. Word embeddings are trained on generic corpora, which limits their direct use for domain specific tasks. Hence, including specific information will improve its utility. Information is added from medical coding data as well as the first level from the hierarchy of ICD-10 medical code. They adapt the CBOW algorithm from the word2vec package. These modified word embeddings give an improvement in f-score by 1% on the 5-fold evaluation on a private medical claims dataset.

An analytical web-based solution is presented in Chawla et al. [25] for detecting adverse drug reactions from user reviews of neurological drugs, as well as visualizing the extent of these reactions and other insights obtained from the reviews. For detection of adverse drug reactions, they train a classifier to label sentences as effective, ineffective, adverse, or none. Eight feature sets based on sentiment scores, TF-IDF vectors, n-grams, etc. are considered and best performance is obtained using TF-IDF vectors and VADER sentiment scores on a OnevsRest classifier. [26] explores argument mining techniques based on machine learning on the same dataset used in

[25], and presents an approach to extract support and attack relations from medical reviews. Each pair of sentences in a review is considered to be a training example, to be classified as either "support," "attack," or "neutral." Seven feature sets based on combinations of structural features [3] and TF-IDF scores for unigrams and bigrams are evaluated on three main classification algorithms: support vector machine, Random Forest classifier, and AdaBoost classifier. The best performance is obtained on a hybrid feature set of structural and TF-IDF scores on an AdaBoost classifier, though class imbalance leads to a low F1 score for the "neutral" category.

Argument mining also finds applications in more specific domains such as legal judgements [27] and scientific literature [28]. Shulayeva et al. [27] aim to classify sentences as principle, fact, or neutral in legal judgements. The nature of the legal data in this case makes a simpler model work with good accuracy, as easily recognizable differences exist (e.g., principles are often stated in present tense while facts are in past tense). The work in [28] aims to create a model that can understand the content and structure of peer reviews.

In this chapter, we narrow our focus on an application of argument mining for the medical domain. Specifically, we consider the task of classifying whether two sentences or phrases from drug reviews present supporting or attacking views, and explore machine learning and ensemble methods to automate the task. An effective system for argument mining must be able to extract consistent relations between sentences, i.e., the relations must make intuitive sense. Considering the challenges that inherently accompany the use of drug reviews, this application can help doctors in taking decisions for a patient but is not a substitute for actual prescriptions.

7.4 METHODOLOGY

7.4.1 Proposed Methodology

Figure 7.1 shows a breakdown of the system design. The system discussed in [25] takes reviews as input from the user. They preprocess the review by removing stop words, punctuations, and performing lemmatization, normalization, and tokenization. They have used TF-IDF features and sentiment scores generated using VADER library as the features for their classification models, which then classifies review sentences into four categories: effective, ineffective, adverse, and other. Based on this categorization, top ranked reviews, pros, and cons are generated for the user. Thus, they have proposed a novel approach for developing a system for classification and analysis of user reviews for drugs used in the treatment of neurological disorders. Their results gave an accuracy of ~75% across three categories – adverse, effective, ineffective. Some deep learning algorithms like LSTM, CNN + LSTM were implemented as well. This gave accuracy of around ~75% with high bias towards the dominant class, i.e., effective category. Finally, they concluded that the machine learning approach is more effective.

In [26], the system takes input in the form of reviews and sentence pairs are formed using the presence of discourse indicators. Machine learning algorithms like SVM, Random Forest, and AdaBoost were used to classify the relationship between two sentences in a pair as either "support," "attack," or "neutral." The number of neutral class examples were fewer as compared to support and attack class

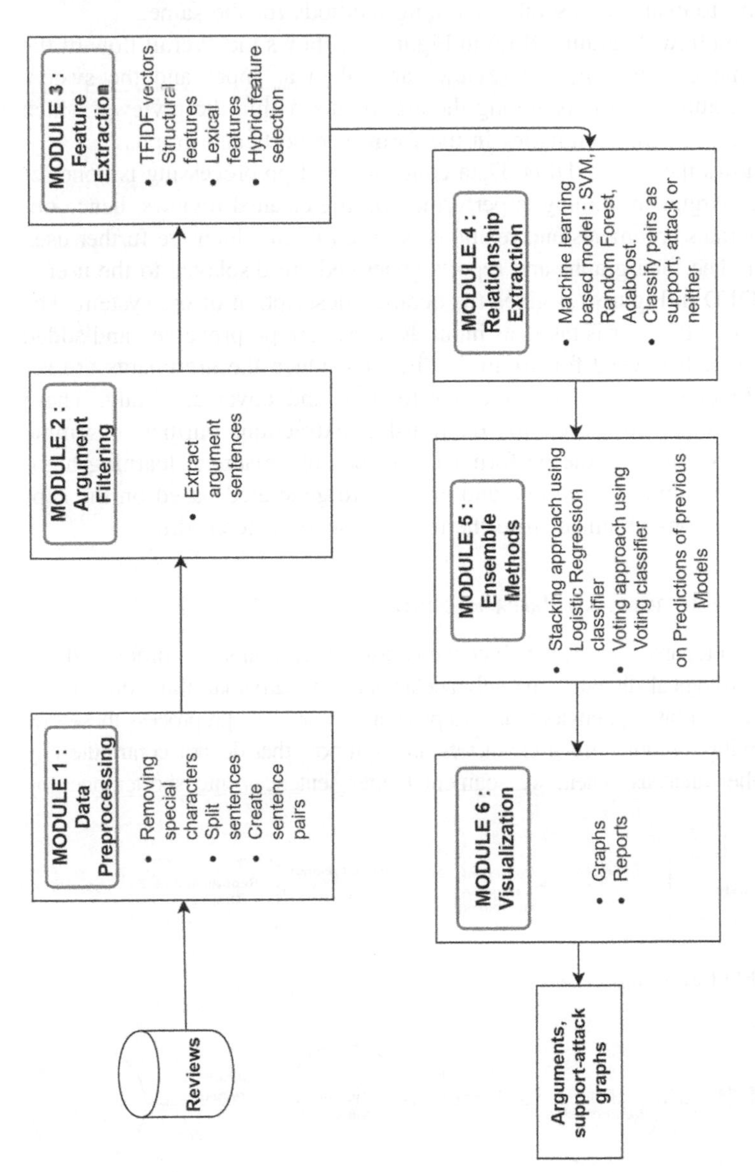

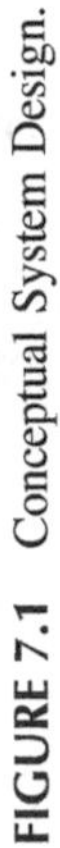
FIGURE 7.1 Conceptual System Design.

examples in the training dataset. This led to a class imbalance which affected the performance of the machine learning algorithms.

We built upon the work presented in [25] and [26], specifically to improve the performance of machine learning classifiers for extracting and visualizing support-attack graphs and to evaluate ensemble learning methods for the same.

The level 0 data flow diagram (DFD) in Figure 7.2 shows the overall flow of the system. The name of the drug and reviews are taken as input and the system generates support-attack relations among the arguments within the reviews, which are further used to develop summaries in the form of reports and graphs.

Figure 7.3 shows the level 1 DFD. Data collection and preprocessing is done for the entered drug. Argument mining is performed on the cleaned reviews, hence obtained. This generates arguments and relations between them which are further used for visualization. The final graphs and reports generated are displayed to the user.

The level 2 DFD in Figure 7.4 gives the detailed description of the system. The review(s) entered by the user is taken as input. Reviews are preprocessed and added to the database which is used for argument filtering. Once the arguments are separated, they are classified as effective, ineffective, and adverse, if any. These classified sentences are now used for relationship extraction. Further, ensemble approach is used to improve the performance of existing machine learning algorithms. The overall summary, reports, and graphs are generated based on the support and attack relations obtained from the reviews of the entered drug.

7.4.2 Data Collection and Preprocessing

We use the corpus prepared in [25] which contains raw reviews on seven different drugs prescribed for neurological disorders, namely acetazolamide, carbamazepine, divalproex, ethosuximide, phenobarbital, phenytoin, and valproic acid. First, we preprocess these raw reviews by removing various special characters and symbols that do not contribute any meaning for further analysis. Then, we segment longer sentences into shorter ones by

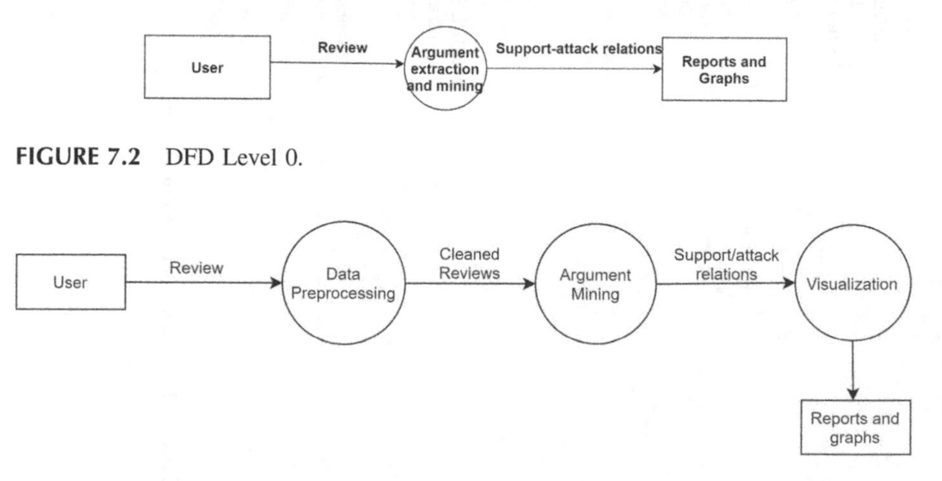

FIGURE 7.2 DFD Level 0.

FIGURE 7.3 DFD Level 1.

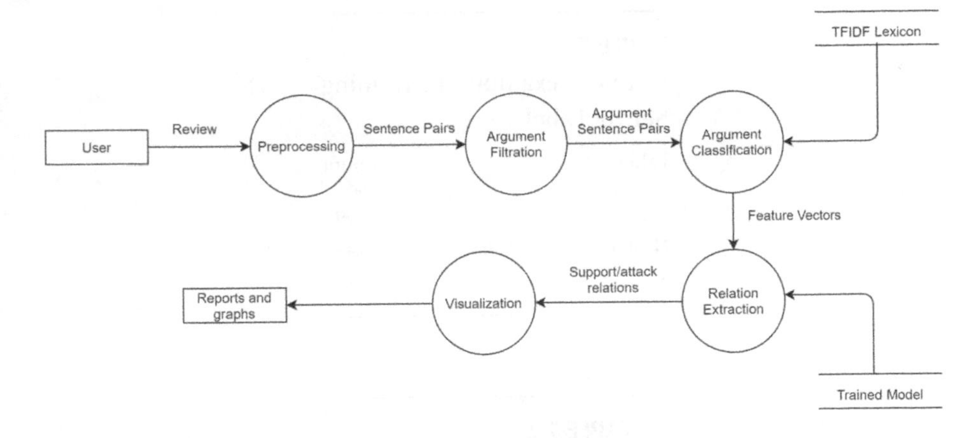

FIGURE 7.4 DFD Level 2.

breaking them on the occurrence of discourse indicators. Discourse indicators are common words that indicate change in flow of logic in a statement. For example, words like yet, however, because, hence, but, etc. Next, we form consecutive sentence pairs as s1 and s2, respectively and then filter out only those pairs containing at least one discourse indicator either in s1 or s2. Then we label those pairs as support, attack, or neutral based on type of discourse indicators both manually as well as programmatically.

To address the problem of overfitting and class imbalance, we consider an additional 474 manually annotated sentence pairs from the review corpus, maintaining the condition that at least one of them contains a discourse indicator. Manual annotation can help incorporate more subtle or indirect examples of support, attack, or neutrality. We add these to the dataset used in [26] and create new training and test sets, with 1,289 and 467 examples in each, respectively. The breakdown of training and test sets are given in Tables 7.1 and 7.2.

For relationship extraction, we train and evaluate classifiers on the training set, considering 80:20 split for training and validation sets. Additionally, the performance of all classifiers is checked on the holdout set of 467 examples, in order to gauge how well each algorithm is able to generalize.

7.4.3 Feature Extraction

In this step, the objective is to create a representation of the data (i.e., sentence pairs) that is suitable for training a machine learning algorithm. The representation must capture accurate information and nuances within the data to render the learning task possible.

We follow the process detailed in [26] for feature extraction. For argument relation extraction, structural features are a good candidate and found to be effective [3,19,26]. For a sentence pair (s1,s2), structural features comprise the number of tokens and punctuations in s1 and s2, as well as their absolute differences.

In addition, we also consider the TF-IDF scores for the top 15,000 unigrams and bigrams for both sentences in a tuple. Structural and TF-IDF scores were found to be the best performing feature sets when used in combination in [26], so we

TABLE 7.1
Count of Examples in Training Set by Label

Label	Count
Attack	599
Neutral	147
Support	543

TABLE 7.2
Count of Examples in Test Set by Label

Label	Count
Attack	222
Neutral	54
Support	191

consider two main feature sets for evaluation (these are analogous to the feature sets "FS6" and "FS7" used in [26]).

- F1: TF-IDF top 15,000 unigrams and bigrams
- F2: Structural features + TF-IDF top 15,000 unigrams and bigrams

9.4.4 Relationship Extraction

For relationship classification, we train machine learning models to classify any pair of sentences or clauses as one of three labels: "support" if the two sentences express supporting views, "attack" if the two sentences express attacking views and "neutral" if there is no particular support or attack relation between them. We consider the following classification algorithms:

- **SVM:** A support-vector machine constructs a hyperplane between the data points which is used for classification, outlier detection, etc. The decision boundary forms the widest margin between separable data points, hence SVMs are also known as maximum margin classifiers.
- **Random Forest:** Random Forest is a supervised ensemble learning algorithm. Random Forest considers multiple decision trees and merges them

together to get a more accurate and stable prediction. It searches for the best feature among a random subset of features rather than searching for the most important feature while splitting a node. This results in a wide diversity that generally results in a better model.

- **AdaBoost:** AdaBoost or Adaptive Boosting is another ensemble-boosting algorithm. It combines various classifiers to increase the accuracy of classifiers. AdaBoost is an iterative ensemble method. It builds a strong classifier by combining multiple poorly performing classifiers to improve the accuracy. The basic concept behind AdaBoost is to set the weights of classifiers and training the data sample in each iteration such that it ensures the accurate predictions of unusual observations. Any machine learning algorithm can be used as a base classifier if it accepts weights on the training set.

We retrain the SVM, Random Forest, and AdaBoost models on new data using ensemble methods and evaluate their performance with old classifiers on unseen data. The comparison of performances is given in Table 7.3.

7.4.5 Ensemble Methods

Ensemble methods are a category of classification algorithms that use multiple models concurrently and combine them to work as a single classifier. Ensemble methods usually improve the accuracy of the machine learning models, and are frequently recommended for out-of-the-box classification. Ensemble learning is a machine learning paradigm where multiple models called "weak learners" are trained to solve the exact same problem and combined to get better results. The assumption is that multiple weak learners give better performance collectively than singular strong learners.

- **Voting ensemble:** In voting, the first step is to create multiple classification/regression models using some training dataset. The base models may be instances of the same algorithm trained on different training subsets, or different algorithms on the same training data or other methods. The final prediction of a voting ensemble is obtained by using voting to combine the individual predictions by the base models. A "hard" voting classifier considers only the majority voted label as the final label, whereas a "soft" voting uses the class probabilities put out by the base models and gives the final label by averaging these probabilities. Voting ensembles do not require the base models to be homogenous. We can train different base learners, e.g., a Random Forest and SVM, and then use the voting ensemble to combine their results. Voting ensembles can improve performance as compared to their base models by making aggregate predictions, thereby reducing the effect of weaknesses of the individual learners.

- **Stacking ensemble:** Stacking or stacked generalization is a multi-tiered or hierarchical ensemble method, wherein the predictions of the base or lower level models are learnt by a meta-model (in effect, we are "stacking" learners

TABLE 7.3
Performance of Classifiers and Comparison with Previous Results

Model	Feature set	Neutral		Support		Attack		F1 (weighted average)	Accuracy (10-fold CV)
		Precision	Recall	Precision	Recall	Precision	Recall		
SVM	f1-o	0.25	0.09	0.92	0.85	0.89	0.97	0.88	89.77%
	f2-o	0.25	0.09	0.94	0.86	0.89	0.98	0.89	89.71%
	f1	0.6	0.58	0.91	0.87	0.95	0.98	0.9	86.32
	f2	0.57	0.5	0.87	0.86	0.96	0.98	0.88	85.56
Random Forest	f1-o	0	0	0.83	0.77	0.82	0.92	0.81	85.24%
	f2-o	0	0	0.84	0.86	0.9	0.95	0.86	85.63%
	f1	0.4	0.15	0.77	0.85	0.88	0.92	0.8	75.16
	f2	0.5	0.15	0.73	0.88	0.89	0.87	0.78	75.56
Ada Boost	f1-o	0.36	0.45	0.94	0.92	0.98	0.97	0.93	95.11%
	f2-o	0.21	0.27	0.93	0.9	0.99	0.99	0.93	95.13%
	f1	0.45	0.5	0.86	0.85	1	0.98	0.89	88.93
	f2	0.45	0.54	0.87	0.83	0.99	0.98	0.88	88.15

on top of each other, hence the name.) The basic idea is to train base classifiers with the training dataset and then generate a new dataset containing the predictions of these models, which is used as training data for a secondary classifier. The meta-learner may be any classification or regression algorithm, such as logistic regression, neural network, etc. Stacking ensemble has the advantage over voting ensemble in that it can map more complex relations and learn better predictions based on the base learners. Stacking ensembles are often heterogeneous, i.e., the base estimators can be different.

We implement a voting and a stacking ensemble by using the best performing models found in the initial training and testing phase for relationship extraction. We implement a hard-voting ensemble based on majority votes. For the stacking ensemble, we use a logistic regression classifier to act as the level 2 classifier and train it based on the predictions made by the three base classifiers. The accuracy of the ensemble classifiers is checked on the holdout set in terms of accuracy and class-wise f1-scores.

7.5 RESULTS AND ANALYSIS

7.5.1 Results

Table 7.3 shows the performance of the three classifiers on the adjusted dataset, compared with that on the initial dataset (represented as "f1-o" or "f2-o"). We obtain the best performance on the SVM with TF-IDF features. Table 7.4 shows the performances of all trained models on the holdout set, while Table 7.5 represents the performances of the two ensemble classifiers on the holdout set. Stacking ensemble gives the best performance with an F1 score of 0.65 and accuracy of 61.45% using TF-IDF scores.

7.5.2 Discussion

Our findings show that while all models clear the majority baseline, the performance of the three base classifiers consistently improves on the holdout set with the addition of structural features, which indicates that hybrid feature sets give better results in predicting argumentative relationships between text. The class imbalance and overfitting problems for the models in [26] are also improved with the addition of manually labeled examples in the extended dataset, as precision and recall for all classifiers improve significantly for the "neutral" category after adjustment.

In addition, the performance of each ensemble model is an improvement over that of the individual classifiers on the holdout set (Table 7.5). The stacking ensemble outperforms the voting ensemble for the dominant classes (support and attack) for both feature sets, though the voting ensemble performs better for "neutral" examples and for recall in the "attack" category, as apparent from the confusion matrices in Figures 7.5 to 7.8.

Neutral pairs remain the most difficult to classify. This can be attributed to the nature of the dataset, as reviews tend to be subjective and are likely to contain argumentative language in favor or against a single topic. The overall accuracy of the system can be improved by adding more data to augment the dataset. Deep

TABLE 7.4
Results of Base Classifiers on Holdout Set

Model	Feature set	Neutral		Support		Attack		F1 (weighted average)	Accuracy (10-fold CV)
		Precision	Recall	Precision	Recall	Precision	Recall		
SVM	f1	0.18	0.46	0.63	0.54	0.85	0.63	0.61	57.60%
	f2	0.2	0.48	0.66	0.56	0.83	0.64	0.62	**58.88%**
Random Forest	f1	0.16	0.06	0.54	0.72	0.68	0.59	0.56	58.24%
	f2	0.11	0.07	0.55	0.68	0.72	0.63	0.58	**58.45%**
Ada Boost	f1	0.15	0.54	0.52	0.35	0.91	0.62	0.55	49.89%
	f2	0.14	0.5	0.53	0.38	0.94	0.61	0.56	**50.10%**

TABLE 7.5
Results Using Ensemble Methods on Holdout Set

Model	Feature set	Neutral		Support		Attack		F1 (weighted average)	Accuracy (10-fold CV)
		Precision	Recall	Precision	Recall	Precision	Recall		
Stacking ensemble	f1	0.19	0.41	0.63	0.7	0.96	0.59	0.65	**61.45%**
	f2	0.18	0.41	0.63	0.66	0.92	0.61	0.64	60.81%
Voting ensemble	f1	0.2	0.46	0.63	0.66	0.94	0.61	0.65	**61.24%**
	f2	0.19	0.5	0.65	0.6	0.91	0.61	0.63	59.31%

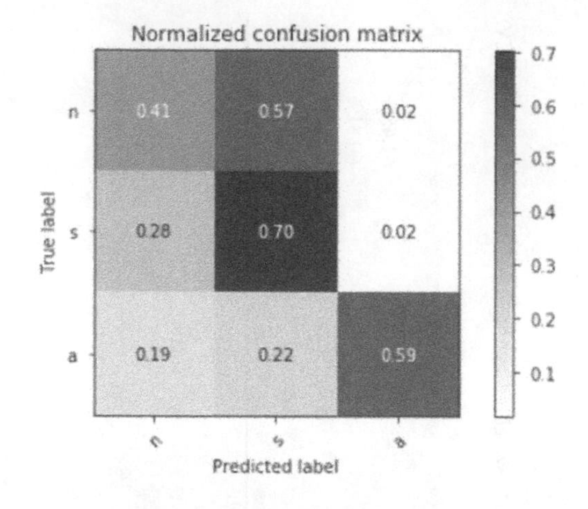

FIGURE 7.5 F1 Stacking Confusion Matrix.

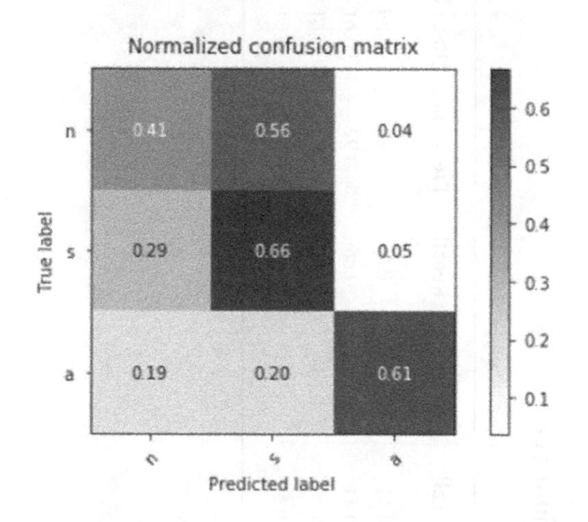

FIGURE 7.6 F2 Stacking Confusion Matrix.

learning methods have also found success in entailment and argumentation tasks [4,13,17], and present a promising direction for further research.

7.5.3 Website

A website has been created which takes input in the form of drug name and either individual reviews or a file containing multiple reviews. The output displayed consists of:

- Detailed report containing the sentence and word count and tense of the words
- Number of support, attack, and neutral pairs and their pie chart
- Graph with sentences in the review as nodes and edges between them indicating support relation (green) or attack relation (red)

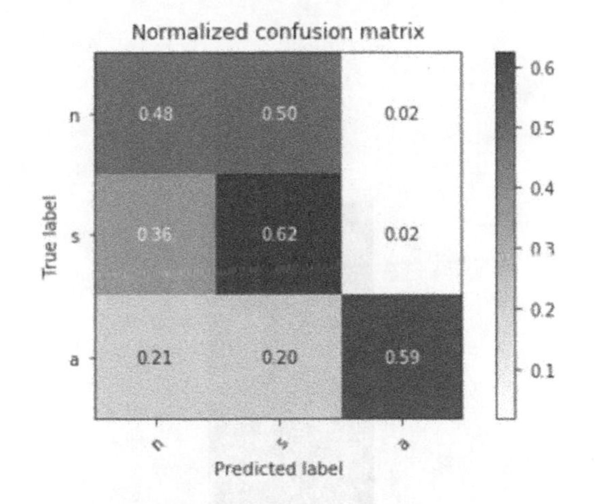

FIGURE 7.7 F1 Voting Confusion Matrix.

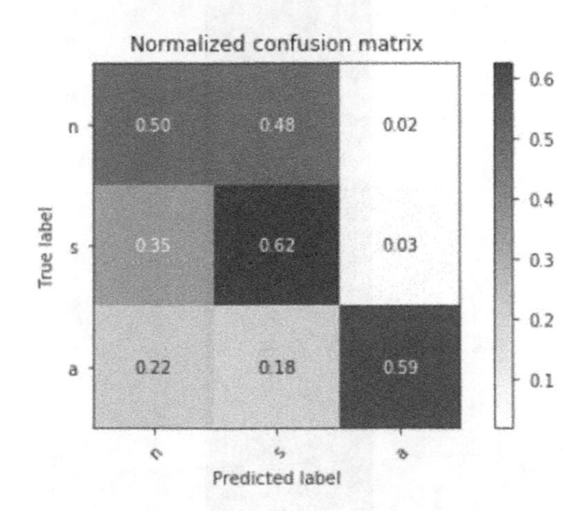

FIGURE 7.8 F2 Voting Confusion Matrix.

- Table containing the sentence pairs and relations between them

The website has been hosted on Heroku which is a cloud Platform as a Service (PaaS). The link for the website is: https://argmining.herokuapp.com/minereview

7.5.4 Argument Graphs and User Interface

The user interface as shown in Figure 7.9 takes the name of a drug and related reviews as input. The input can be either a single review (Figure 7.10) or a bunch of them consolidated into a CSV file (Figure 7.11). The application further pre-processes this data and generates a detailed report. This includes the word and sentence count of the reviews and the predominant tenses. Finally, the argument relation pairs are displayed along with their connectivity graphs.

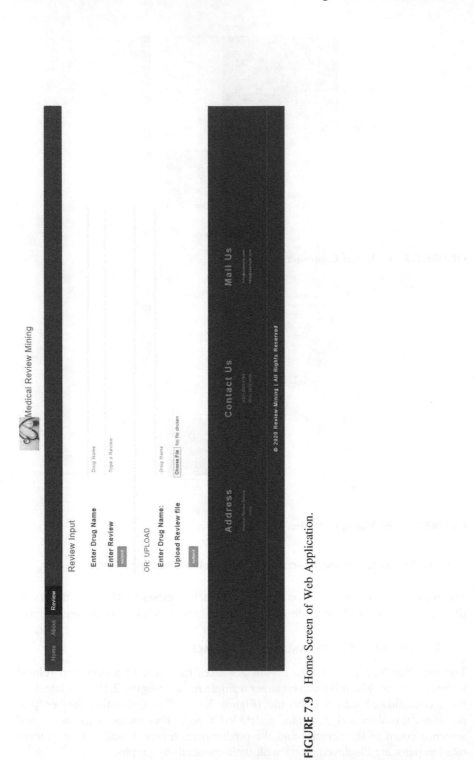

FIGURE 7.9 Home Screen of Web Application.

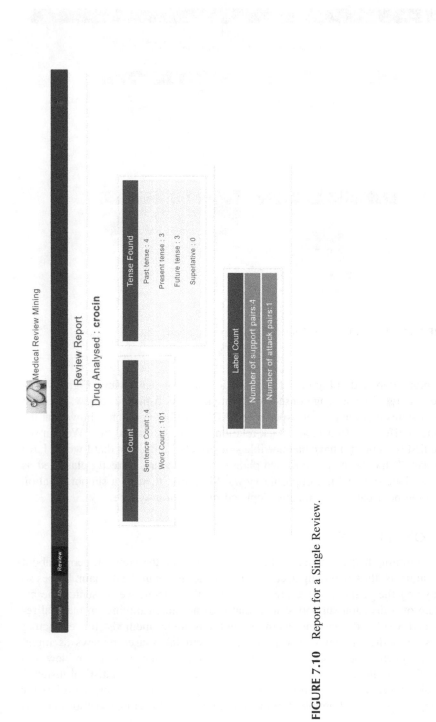

FIGURE 7.10 Report for a Single Review.

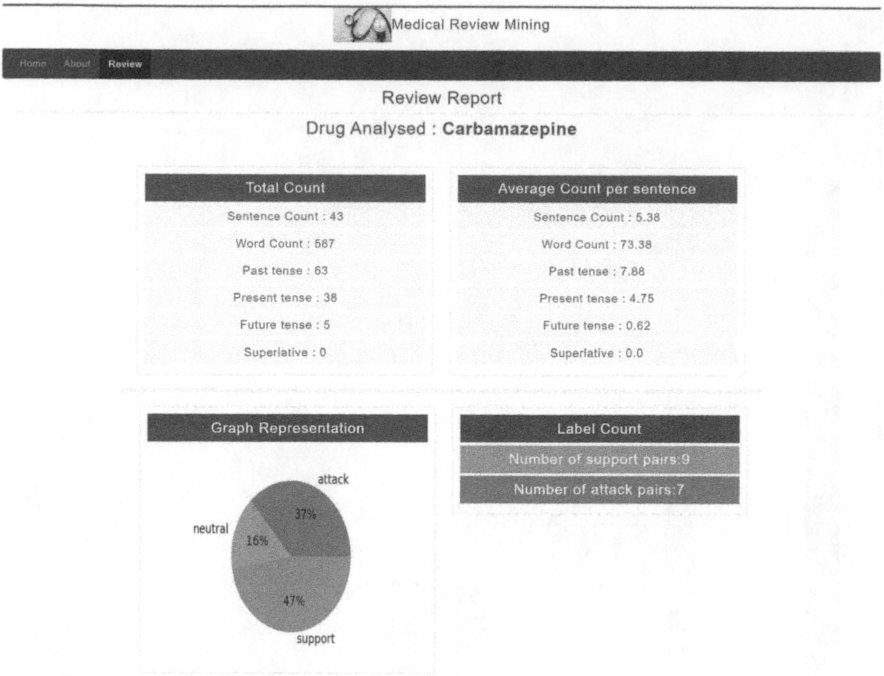

FIGURE 7.11 Report Generated for Carbamazepine Reviews.

The graph depicted in Figure 7.12 is done for an unlabeled review (Figure 7.13). It represents relations among consecutive sentence pairs from the review. The first argument states that the patient experienced ADRs while the second shows that the medicine is effective. Hence, an attack relation, denoted by a red line. We can see that the first sentence ("I have had horrible side effects… episodes that I would have almost daily") has been split into two phrases, and they are correctly classified as attacking, since they exhibit opposing views. Similarly, there is a support relation between the next pair of arguments, depicted by a light gray line.

7.6 CONCLUSION

Argument mining helps us ascertain the reasoning behind the views of people about various subjects, thus providing accurate understanding about the domain. It does so by analyzing the semantic structure of text. In this chapter, we presented the architecture of a decision support system that uses argument mining on medical reviews, and explored machine learning and ensemble methods for extracting relations from drug reviews. The proposed system takes user reviews as input, extracts supporting or attacking relationships among sentences in the review and displays these in the form of argument graphs, along with other statistical insights. Our results improve upon existing work in building machine learning classifiers for extracting support-attack graphs from unstructured text. Ensemble methods helped

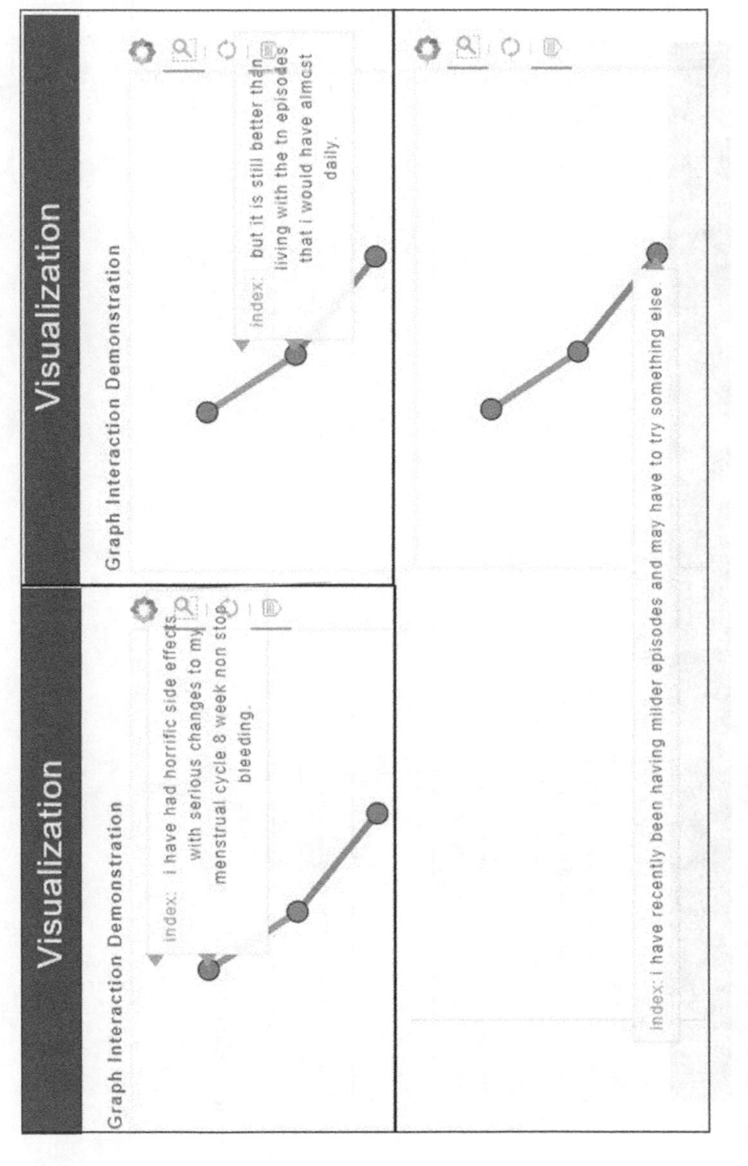

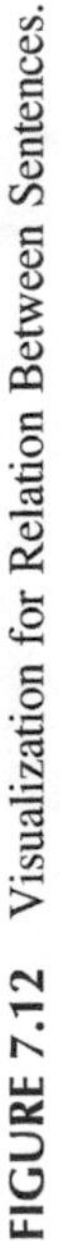

FIGURE 7.12 Visualization for Relation Between Sentences.

List of Sentence Pairs

Sentence 1	Sentence 2	Relation
this is a medicine which will cure ur headache intially for 5 or6 times.	but after that ur body get used to it simply an adiction drug which can make ur body adicted to this drug.	attack
but after that ur body get used to it simply an adiction drug which can make ur body adicted to this drug.	my friend work in a private company and used to take medicine regulary and more often crocin.	support
my friend work in a private company and used to take medicine regulary and more often crocin.	because of work pressure.	support
because of work pressure.	now he get stick to this medicin and get adicted now he has to take crocin in regular interval.	support
so guys i will suggest u not to take crocin more regularly only take.	when its very imergent and necessary to take it	support

FIGURE 7.13 Sentences and the Relation Between Them.

improve the overall performance of our base models. Further improvements in performance and quality of mined arguments can be obtained by using data augmentation, as well as exploring alternative learning methods like deep learning.

Such a system can potentially assist medical practitioners to identify commonly raised pros and cons associated with drugs from a large bulk of user reviews, and provide a deeper-level insight into public opinion. This information can assist medical practitioners and analysts to make sound decisions while prescribing drugs and spread awareness among patients about the new characteristics concerning the medicines.

REFERENCES

[1]. L. Elezabeth, and V. P. Mishra, "Big Data Mining Methods in Medical Applications." In Medical Big Data and Internet of Medical Things: Advances, Challenges and Applications. A. E. Hassanien, N. Dey, S. Borra (eds). Boca Raton, Florida: CRC Press/Taylor & Francis, 2018, pp. 1–24.

[2]. S. Abbas, and H. Sawamura, "A First Step Towards Argument Mining and Its Use in Arguing Agents and ITS." In Knowledge-Based Intelligent Information and Engineering Systems. I. Lovrek, R. J. Howlett, L. C. Jain (eds). Berlin, Heidelberg: Springer, 2008.

[3]. C. Stab, and I. Gurevych, "Identifying Argumentative Discourse Structures in Persuasive Essays." In Proceedings of the 2014 Conference on Empirical Methods in Natural Language Processing (EMNLP), pp. 46–56, 2014.

[4]. O. Cocarascu, and F. Toni, "Combining Deep Learning and Argumentative Reasoning for the Analysis of Social Media Textual Content Using Small Data Sets." Computational Linguistics, vol. 44, no. 4, pp. 833–858, 2018. Available: 10.1162/coli_a_00338.

[5]. F. Gobbo, M. Benini, and J. Wagemans, "Annotation with Adpositional Argumentation." Intelligenza Artificiale, vol. 13, no. 2, pp. 155–172, 2020.

[6]. J. Wagemans, "Constructing a Periodic Table of Arguments." In Argumentation, Objectivity, and Bias: Proceedings of the 11th International Conference of the Ontario Society for the Study of Argumentation (OSSA). P. Bondy, L. Benacquista (eds). Windsor, ON: OSSA, pp. 1–12, 18–21, 2016. Available: 10.2139/ssrn.2769833.

[7]. W. Sun, Z. Cai, Y. Li, F. Liu, S. Fang, and G. Wang, "Data Processing and Text Mining Technologies on Electronic Medical Records: A Review." Journal of Healthcare Engineering, vol. 2018, pp. 4302425, 2018.

[8]. A. Peldszus, and M. Stede, "From Argument Diagrams to Argumentation Mining in Texts: A Survey." IJCINI, vol. 7, pp. 1–31, 2013.

[9]. R. Levy, Y. Bilu, D. Hershcovich, E. Aharoni, and N. Slonim, "Context Dependent Claim Detection." In Proceedings of COLING 2014, the 25th International Conference on Computational Linguistics: Technical Papers, pp. 1489–1500, 2014.

[10]. R. Rinott, L. Dankin, C. A. Perez, M. M. Khapra, E. Aharoni, and N. Slonim, "Show Me Your Evidence-An Automatic Method for Context Dependent Evidence Detection." In Proceedings of the 2015 Conference on Empirical Methods in Natural Language Processing, pp. 440–450, 2015.

[11]. E. Aharoni, A. Polnarov, T. Lavee, D. Hershcovich, R. Levy, R. Rinott, D. Gutfreund, and N. Slonim, "A Benchmark Dataset for Automatic Detection of Claims and Evidence in the Context of Controversial Topics." In Proceedings of the First Workshop on Argumentation Mining, pp. 64–68, 2014.

[12]. R. Levy, S. Gretz, B. Sznajder, S. Hummel, R. Aharonov, and N. Slonim, "Unsupervised Corpus–Wide Claim Detection." In Proceedings of the 4th Workshop on Argument Mining, 2017. Available: 10.18653/v1/w17-5110.

[13]. R. Levy, Y. Bilu, D. Hershcovich, E. Aharoni, and N. Slonim, "Towards an Argumentative Content Search Engine Using Weak Supervision." In Proceedings of the 27th International Conference on Computational Linguistics, pp. 2066–2081, 2018.
[14]. T. Mikolov, S. Ilya, C. Kai, C. Greg, and D. Jeffrey, "Distributed Representations of Words and Phrases and their Compositionality." Advances in Neural Information Processing Systems, vol. 26, 2013.
[15]. R. Bar-Haim, I. Bhattacharya, F. Dinuzzo, A. Saha, and N. Slonim, "Stance Classification of Context-Dependent Claims." EACL, no. 1, pp. 251–261, 2017.
[16]. S. Mirkin, G. Moshkowich, M. Orbach, L. Kotlerman, Y. Kantor, T. Lavee, M. Jacovi, Y. Bilu, R. Aharonov, and N. Slonim, "Listening Comprehension Over Argumentative Content." In Proceedings of the 2018 Conference on Empirical Methods in Natural Language Processing, pp. 719–724, 2018.
[17]. M. Gleize, E. Shnarch, L. Choshen, L. Dankin, G. Moshkowich, R. Aharonov, and N. Slonim, "Are You Convinced? Choosing the More Convincing Evidence with a Siamese Network." In Proceedings of the 57th Annual Meeting of the Association for Computational Linguistics, pp. 967–976, 2019.
[18]. C. Stab, J. Daxenberger, C. Stahlhut, T. Miller, B. Schiller, C. Tauchmann, S. Eger, and I. Gurevych, "ArgumenText: Searching for Arguments in Heterogeneous Sources." In Proceedings of the 2018 Conference of the North American Chapter of the Association for Computational Linguistics: Demonstrations, pp. 21–25, 2018.
[19]. B. Aker, A. Sliwa, Y. Ma, R. Lui, N. Borad, S. Ziyaei, and M. Ghobadi, "What Works and What Does Not: Classifier and Feature Analysis for Argument Mining." In Proceedings of the 4th Workshop on Argument Mining, pp. 91–96, 2017.
[20]. J. Lawrence, and C. Reed, "Combining Argument Mining Techniques." In Proceedings of the 2nd Workshop on Argumentation Mining, pp. 127–136, 2015.
[21]. S. Hochreiter, and J. Schmidhuber, "Long Short-Term Memory." Neural Computation, vol. 9, no. 8, pp. 1735–1780, 1997.
[22]. J. Pennington, R. Socher, and C. Manning, "Glove: Global Vectors for Word Representation." EMNLP, vol. 14, pp. 1532–1543, 2014. Available: 10.3115/v1/D14-1162.
[23]. K. Noor, A. Hunter, and A. Mayer, "Analysis of Medical Arguments from Patient Experiences Expressed on the Social Web." In Proceedings of the International Conference on Industrial, Engineering and Other Applications of Applied Intelligent Systems, pp. 285–294, 2017.
[24]. K. Patel, D. Patel, M. Golakiya, Bhattacharyya P., and N. Birari, "Adapting Pre-trained Word Embeddings for Use in Medical Coding." BioNLP, vol. 2017, pp. 302–306, 2017.
[25]. D. Chawla, D. Mohnani, V. Sawlani, S. Varma, and S. Khedkar, "Drug Review Analytics of Neurological Disorders." In Proceedings of the 2019 International Conference on Nascent Technologies in Engineering (ICNTE), pp. 1–3, 2019.
[26]. A. Bhattacharya, K. Kumbhar, P. Borwankar, A. Mendes, and S. Khedkar, "Argument Mining for Medical Reviews." International Journal of Future Generation Communication and Networking, vol. 13, no. 1s, pp. 226–233, 2020.
[27]. O. Shulayeva, A. Siddharthan, and A. Wyner, "Recognizing Cited Facts and Principles in Legal Judgements." In Proceedings of the Artificial Intelligence for Justice Workshop at the 22nd European Conference on Artificial Intelligence (ECAI 2016), 2016.
[28]. X. Hua, M. Nikolov, N. Badugu, and L. Wang, "Argument Mining for Understanding Peer Reviews." 2019. arXiv preprint arXiv:1903.10104.

8 Augmented Reality Systems and Haptic Devices for Needle Insertion Medical Training

Cléber Gimenez Corrêa, Claiton de Oliveira, and Silvio Ricardo Rodrigues Sanches
Universidade Tecnológica Federal do Paraná (UTFPR), Cornélio Procópio, Brazil

CONTENTS

8.1 INTRODUCTION

Deaths due to medical errors are reported in many countries. In the United States, for example, medical errors are the third leading cause of death of the population, being that the first and the second are cancer and heart diseases, respectively (Makary and Daniel, 2016). In the UK, research shows that hospitals have high expenses due to medical errors (Iacobucci, 2014). Thus, medical training becomes an important aspect, affecting the economy, policy, and quality of life of the citizens.

The revolution in digital information has led to rapid advancements in the medical systems (Hassanien et al., 2018). Computer systems can be tools to provide training, simulating situations found in the medical procedures to the student to acquire knowledge and sensorimotor skills. These computer systems can reduce

DOI: 10.1201/9781003198796-8

risks for patients (Akhtar et al., 2014; Coles et al., 2011a,b,c), increase the apprentices' certainty, since the procedures can be performed in patients after acquiring experience (Shakil et al., 2012; O'Neill et al., 2011; Lambden and Martin, 2011), and enable the execution of automated user performance assessment, creating metrics, measures, and criteria for analyzing knowledge and skills (Willis et al., 2014). These systems can provide several levels of training, with different situations and degrees of difficulty that can happen during the procedure (Ullrich and Kuhlen, 2012). They can also minimize the cost of creating and keeping physical laboratories with objects consisting of animals or cadavers for training (Gomoll et al., 2007; Balcombe, 2004).

There are anatomical differences between animals and human beings (Aboud et al., 2004), as well as ethical and of preparation issues involving the use of these animals in the training (Coles et al., 2011a; Balcombe, 2004). Although cadavers offer physical presence when compared to the simulation generated only with computers, they have physiological differences in relation to living organisms, such as arterial pulse (Jaung et al., 2011). Another advantage of computer-based simulations is the high number of possible training repetitions without the wearing of materials, as is the case of training using cadavers (Grechenig et al., 1999).

Most of the three-dimensional (3D) systems used for medical training are Virtual Reality (VR) systems (Corrêa et al., 2019). Although the training environments that use VR offer facilities for the practice of various tasks, these environments consist of a simulation of reality (Wang and Dunston, 2007). This can result in well-trained specialists in these simulators where the graphic quality of the synthetic environment rarely reaches a high level of realism. In AR systems, the training user can view the real environment, which brings the scenes found in the training environment closer to the real situations. According to Botden and Jakimowicz (2009), medical training environments that use VR do not present realistic tactile feedback. On the other hand, simulators using AR retain realistic tactile feedback and, for this reason, can provide a more accurate evaluation of the performances in training. Many studies show the effectiveness of AR environments in medical training (Chaballout et al., 2016). Shinde et al. (2020) mention the potential of AR in different medical training and how this technology can contribute to the health area, integrating, for example, with the Internet of Things technology.

Training based on VR and AR, especially for the acquisition of motor skills, involves the use of the so-called haptic devices, which provide touch feedback, allowing to develop systems with the combination of graphic, sound, and tactile resources, increasing the realism during the training with tools.

Needle insertion is an interesting task to study because it is present in many medical procedures, such as anesthesia, biopsy, suture, injection, spinal intervention, and other radiological interventions. The performance of some medical procedures occurs with the support of images, and in certain cases, a sequence of images, from computed tomography, ultrasound, requiring manual skill while observing the anatomical structures and the needle in a monitor (Sutherland et al., 2011, 2013). In other procedures, the medical professional must manipulate a needle and a probe, which captures these images in real time to show in a monitor.

There are procedures that consist of palpation and needle insertion tasks, which must be performed simultaneously by a medical professional (Coles et al., 2011b). There are also procedures without visual support to guide the professional. In this case, the medical professional performs the procedure with only the knowledge of anatomy and tactile sensation (Corrêa et al., 2017). Other important questions in the insertion task involve the size of the needle, whether it is flexible or rigid and the shape of the needle tip, depending on the procedure to be trained (Corrêa et al., 2019).

Simulation is a safe way of medical procedures training, for patients and future professionals, preventing errors and injuries. AR systems with haptic devices are promising technologies that allow simulations of these procedures. In the past decade, there has been an increase in the number of studies that use haptic devices to interact with computer systems (Varalakshmi et al., 2012), including AR. Then, we analyzed the most relevant works to identify the most suitable devices and procedures, which require needle insertion, which can be simulated using these devices to allow interaction in an AR system.

This chapter presents research on training in medical procedures that involve needle insertion through computer systems based on Augmented Reality (AR) and haptic devices that allow simulating different scenarios to practice before the actual performance.

This chapter is organized as follows: Section 8.2 presents the concepts about AR, including main characteristics of the AR-based systems; Section 8.3 addresses the haptic devices, presenting their characteristics; Section 8.4 describes studies about AR-based systems and haptic devices for medical procedures training in which the needle insertion task is relevant; Section 8.5 presents an analysis of the studies cited in the previous section; Section 8.6 shows the challenges, trends, and opportunities in the context of AR systems and haptic devices for medical training in needle insertion; and, finally, this chapter concludes with Section 8.7.

8.2 AUGMENTED REALITY (AR)

AR systems have been present in the computing world for a few decades. Research in this area has as its basic objective to increase user perception and interaction with the real world by supplementing reality with 3D virtual objects that seem to coexist in the same space (Azuma, 2004). According to Azuma (2004), utopia is the creation of an environment in which the user cannot distinguish the real world from the virtually augmented.

Some components considered important in AR systems are the devices used to view or interact with these systems. Some decades ago, the definition of AR-associated applications with the use of Head-Mounted Displays (HMDs); however, this became very restrictive, and a good part of the systems of the time would not fall under this definition.

Azuma (1997) presented a much more comprehensive idea to define AR systems based on three essential characteristics: (i) the combination of something real and virtual, that is, the coexistence of real and virtual elements in three dimensions, with a predominance of real elements, (ii) human–computer interaction in real time, and (iii) precise alignment and synchronization of 3D virtual objects with the real environment, called 3D registration. Thus, the characterization of AR systems does not link them to any type of specific device.

Despite this, the equipment used for visualization and interaction remains an important component in applications. The display device, for example, often determines the user's level of immersion in the augmented environment. In simpler systems, which can run on desktops, laptops, tablets, or smartphones, most of the time, the user visualizes the enlarged environment through the device's screen. Normally, systems capture the real environment using a camera, process the captured real scene, add virtual objects (graphic rendering), and present all the content on the screen for visualization. In this case, the level of immersion may be limited. On the other hand, systems equipped with glasses or HMDs can provide a higher level of immersion to the user, who may feel inside the environment.

The interaction with an AR application can also be performed through different devices. Conventional equipment, such as a keyboard and mouse, are common ways of interacting with systems running on desktops or laptops. Platforms such as tablets and smartphones, for example, usually enable interaction by touching the screen.

In most AR applications, virtual objects are inserted into the scene overlaid with markers, which are highlighted designs or marks, most often printed on plain paper. Such markers are placed in the real environment and are identified by the applications when the scene is processed. In this way, these virtual objects are aligned with the real environment, as they are rendered over the marker and can be moved through these marks. More sophisticated systems, however, exploit characteristics of the real environment (e.g., colors and textures) to align and enable interaction with virtual objects. In this case, artificially created markers are not necessary.

In interaction, haptic devices, for example, have been used to allow users tactile feedback, when interacting with virtual elements of the scene. Thus, besides the environment with real and virtual objects displayed graphically on the screen or in the HMD, it is possible to provide a tactile sensation in the interaction with virtual objects.

The application areas of AR are constantly expanding. In the past decades, new projects are constantly being presented in engineering, equipment maintenance, training, as well as collaborative applications for video conferencing, or those focused on entertainment. There are also AR systems developed for educational purposes such as environmental sciences, humanities, arts, and chemistry (Tang et al., 2020).

Besides these areas, the literature presents many other AR projects focused on medicine. Recent studies show that there is an increasing number of applications in this area. According to Tang et al. (2020), these systems are a new paradigm in medical training (Tang et al., 2020). These 3D objects can be constructed from computed tomography and ultrasound images. It is possible to verify, on a real scale, anatomical structures (tissues, blood vessels, nerves, etc.) superimposed on a real mannequin or patient, checking where the needle can pass to reach a target region, because the medical professional can see through the patient's body, avoiding adjacent vital regions and planning the procedure (Hassanien et al., 2018).

In addition to AR technologies, various medical procedures use training simulations with haptic interfaces, including needle insertion specialty (Coles et al., 2011a).

8.3 HAPTIC DEVICES

The introduction of the word "haptic" in the literature happened in the early twentieth century when psychophysicists used it to describe studies that addressed perception and manipulation based on human touch (Salisbury et al., 2004). From the 1990s, the word started to be used in the field of computing with its current meaning. According to Salisbury et al. (2004), haptics refers to touch interactions (physical contact) that occur for the purpose of perception or manipulation of objects. These interactions occur, for example, between a human hand and a virtual object using a haptic interface device.

The haptic devices allow the development of applications with tactile and force feedback. Tactile feedback devices are those that offer interaction with the nerve endings of the skin that indicate the shape, warmth, and texture of objects. Force feedback devices interact with muscles and tendons, giving the user the feeling of applying a force in the opposite direction. Tactile and force feedback brings information about the weight of the object and its consistency/stiffness.

According to Corrêa et al. (2019), haptic devices that are developed for specific purposes in medical projects can be found in the literature. There are also commercial devices of general use and force capture devices used to analyze the properties or parameters of real tissues or organs.

Commercial haptic devices are often used in medical applications where tactile and force feedback are important features for the application. In applications that simulate needle insertion, such devices may be ergonomically inadequate since the part handled by the user does not have the same shape as the actual simulated instrument (Corrêa et al., 2019). To minimize this problem, it is possible to replace parts of some equipment to make it more ergonomic. On the other hand, there are devices that can be easily integrated into the systems due to the availability of software libraries and plugins developed by the suppliers themselves or by the scientific community. Many researchers have started combining AR and haptic interaction to allow users to see and touch digital information embedded in the real environment (Eck et al., 2015).

The devices of this kind have certain characteristics, such as workspace size, that is the maximum range for handling the device styles in a 3D space, measured in millimeters (mm); the number of degrees of freedom of movement (DoF), for example, to perform translation movements in the three axes (x, y, and z) are necessary three degrees of freedom; the number of degrees of freedom of force feedback (DoFF), to provide force feedback in several axes; the maximum force of feedback, analyzed in Newtons (N). These characteristics impact the price of the device and the possibilities for human–computer interaction. Depending on medical procedure, one degree of freedom is enough for simulating the needle behavior. However, to reach a high realism in needle insertion tasks, it is desired a simulation with six degrees of freedom of movement, allowing translation and rotation movements in the three axes.

TABLE 8.1
Examples of Commercial Devices and Their Characteristics (Adapted from Coles et al., 2011a; Corrêa et al., 2019)

Device	Workspace – x, y, and z axes (mm)	Force maximum (N)	DoF	DoFF	Price – Euros
Geomagic Touch	160 × 120 × 70	3.3	6	3	2,000
Phantom Premium 1.5*	191 × 267 × 381	8.5	6	3 or 6	24,000 to 51,000
Novint Falcon	101 × 101 × 101	9	3	3	200
Touch X	160 × 130 × 130	7.9	6	3	11,000
Delta*	360 × 360 × 300	20	3 or 6	3 or 6	22,000 to 40,000
Cyberforce	304 × 304 × 495	8.8	6	3	45,000
Virtuose 6D Desktop	129 × 120 × 120	10	6	6	30,000
Omega*	160 × 160 × 110	3, 6 or 7	6	3	14,000 to 24,000

Notes
* There are different versions of the same device.

In Table 8.1, examples of commercial devices used in simulators for training in the medical systems, including AR and VR systems, are presented. The devices Geomagic Touch and Touch X were previously known as SensAble Phantom Omni and Phantom Desktop, respectively.

The haptic sensations in the AR systems can be provided using electro-mechanical devices, especially force feedback equipment, with sensors and actuators, that can be handled by users to move virtual needles. Additionally, these sensations can be provided using artificial real objects, to imitate anatomical structures, such as bones and soft tissues, and the needle.

Geomagic Touch is an electromechanical device with purpose in kinesthetic feedback widely used in insertion medical training (Jarillo-Silva et al., 2009). Recent research shows that this model is the most used in applications of this type due to its cost-benefit (Corrêa et al., 2019).

Geomagic Touch has six DoF and three DoFF and reaches 3.3 N of force maximum. The force maximum is important because in some simulations the needle during puncture will pass by soft tissues, but it can not pass by bones or other rigid structures. Figure 8.1 shows a Geomagic Touch device.

Although this device offers interesting characteristics for simulating needle insertion, especially the type with six DoFF, its cost is higher than the Geomagic Touch. This device has two types, with differences in DoFF characteristics (one type with 3 and another with 6 degrees). Its workspace is larger than the workspaces of the devices Geomagic Touch and Novint Falcon; six DoF (similar to Geomagic

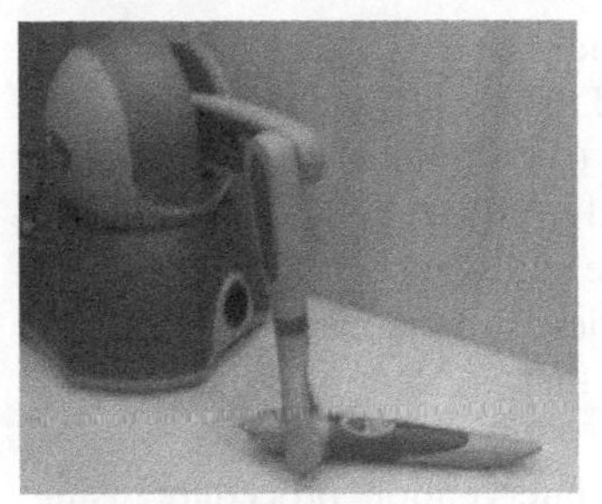

FIGURE 8.1 Geomagic Touch Device.

Touch and higher number of degrees than the Novint Falcon); 8.5 N of force maximum (higher than the Geomagic Touch and lower than the Novint Falcon).

One type of the Phantom Premium 1.5 has six DoFF (higher number than Geomagic Touch and Novint Falcon), allowing to simulate force feedback in three axes of the 3D space for the needle. Considering its characteristics, the cost of this device is high, especially the type with six DoFF.

Novint Falcon device has the lowest price and a higher maximum force than the Geomagic Touch and Premium 1.5 (Table 8.1). However, this device was not commonly used in needle insertion applications. The probable explanation for this is that this equipment has only three degrees of freedom of movement. This limitation makes it difficult to perform the needle insertion task, especially rotation movements. Despite this limitation, the literature contains some VR systems that use the Novint Falcon to simulate certain procedures with needle insertion tasks (Corrêa et al., 2019).

8.4 AR SYSTEMS WITH HAPTIC DEVICES

There are various types of simulators for needle insertion training that aim realism, based on VR, tangible objects, and AR. VR systems create synthetic environments, allowing real-time human–computer interaction and 3D visualization, using conventional (video monitors) or nonconventional (HMDs or special glasses) devices. Tangible objects are physical elements that simulate needle and anatomical structures, with no virtual objects. AR simulators focus on real environments with virtual elements, and real-time 3D human–computer interaction (Corrêa et al., 2019).

We can find several AR systems with haptic devices over the past decade in the literature. In this section, we described some works, highlighting the procedure, target body region, haptic device used, and information about user evaluation such as the number of participants (beginners and experts) in the experiments. The user evaluation is an important step in the development of computer systems for medical training, considering the participants in the experiments and their levels of experience.

In the context, the procedure is the medical intervention in which there is the needle insertion task. In this task, a professional performs 3D movements (position and rotation), inside and outside of the patient's body, puncturing (contacting and cutting the tissues) and extracting the needle. Target body region is the main part of the body, where the needle will be inserted during the procedure. The AR systems must basically simulate these target body regions and the needle, including features (stiffness, volume, viscosity, format) and behaviors (deformation and movements independent of the user's action) of each region and needle type. Participants are users that took part in the evaluation experiments. The participants can be experts or beginners, in which experts are physicians with experience in the medical procedure of interest; and beginners are students or residents that are learning the medical procedure of interest.

In 2011, a study about the invasive minimally intervention procedure using needle insertion was published. The procedure focused on the femoral artery (target body region), and skills of palpation with hand and needle insertion were required. A system was developed with three haptic devices: two Novint Falcon for palpation and a Geomagic Touch for needle insertion. The system consisted in a workspace, where the devices were hidden below the blue sheet, and used a Liquid Crystal Display (LCD) and a camera mounted above the devices to capture the hands of the users. Another camera, of low resolution and side mounted, is used in the shadowing effect of the user's hands. The user visualized his/her hands, the patient covered by a blue sheet and the real needle through LCD display, removing from the scene other parts of the workspace (Coles et al., 2011b).

The Novint Falcon devices were rotated through 90 degrees, coupled together and mounted with an additional pneumatically actuated tactile end effector for simulating femoral artery pulse; and the device Geomagic Touch was modified, fitting a real needle hub (a part of the device's arm was removed) (Coles et al., 2011c). A user evaluation was made with seven experts, using a questionnaire to measure the realism of the system (Coles et al., 2011b).

The next two studies were conducted for the same research group, showing the improvement of the training of the spinal intervention procedure. Thus, the target body region was the spine and the haptic device was the Phantom Premium 1.5-A, a commercial device, like the devices employed in the previous study. The system used a MicronTracker2 camera and a monitor. In the first study of this research group, the system used fiducial markers in a box, in which the box had the upper part opened, allowing the haptic device access to its interior, similar to a needle that punctures the skin, reaching anatomical internal structures close to spine and the vertebrae. MicronTracker2 camera uses stereoscopic vision to detect and track the markers (Sutherland et al., 2011).

In the second publication of this group, in the year 2013, the researchers used a real mannequin with a part of the human body, containing external (torso) and internal (spine) regions, and the fiducial markers were positioned in a mannequin (left side of the mannequin). Additionally, a real object was used for simulating a probe. Radiological intervention can use images from ultrasound, captured through the probe, to help the medical professionals (Sutherland et al., 2013).

The system-generated virtual objects that represent anatomical structures, such as ligament and soft tissue, to overlay the real objects, that represented some vertebrae and skin Images from computed tomography were used to build these objects (Sutherland et al., 2013). Image-processing techniques can be used to build 3D virtual objects from computed tomography, ultrasound and magnetic resonance.

A user evaluation was made with four radiology residents that had experience with needle insertion tasks, three students, and three technicians with experience in viewing ultrasound images. A questionnaire was applied and was divided into three parts: system functionality, graphical user interface, and haptic feedback (Sutherland et al., 2013).

An optometry procedure, whose target body region is one of the eyes, was also studied, with the publication in the year 2013. In this case, a Geomagic Touch was used by researchers for developing the systems. They also used a slit lamp instrument, similar to the equipment used in the real procedure to the professional to visualize the eye, a real mannequin that represented the human head, a fiducial in the front of this mannequin, and a high-definition webcam to capture the marker and add virtual object (Wei et al., 2013).

The 3D workspace of the Geomagic Touch is small compared to other haptic devices (e.g., Phantom Premium 1.5). To overcome this limitation, the researchers changed to the x and z axes, since the available space of the device's x axis in millimeters is larger than the z axis. Thus, the space of movement between the user and the virtual eye was increased. A user assessment was conducted, with the presence of five beginners, divided in subjective and objective evaluation. The participants asked a questionnaire after using the system, and information was captured during human–computer interaction, such as time taken to complete the task, the number of contacts with the eye and severe operational errors (Wei et al., 2013).

Another procedure simulated using an AR-based system and haptic sensation was the urethrovesical anastomosis, and the target body region is the urethra. This work, published in the year 2015, dealt with a user assessment with 52 participants from three different medical centers, that performed tasks in inanimate real objects to simulate anatomical structures, using the daVinci Surgical System. This system is a commercial robot for surgery that is controlled by a physician (Chowriappa et al., 2015). Coles et al. (2011a) mentioned that medical professionals from different hospitals can carry out the same procedure in different ways, based on local experiences.

The evaluation was conducted using a questionnaire and certain measures. The measures were information about needle position, needle driving, suture placement, and tissue manipulation. In this study, the researchers combined subjective and objective evaluations in their experiments. The questionnaire applied for cognition assessment was National Aeronautics and Space Administration – Task Load Index (NASA TLX); and two scores were also applied: Global Evaluative Assessment of Robotic Skills (GEARS) score and an urethrovesical anastomosis score, allowing to assess robotic and procedural skills, respectively (Chowriappa et al., 2015).

Robotic systems had been used in medical procedures to obtain precision and reduce risks to the patients. A literature review about robotic spine surgery and AR systems, including VR systems, can be found in Vadalà et al. (2020), mentioning the importance of information superimposed in the real world to help the medical professionals. Similar to the first study presented, in which the target body region was an artery, other studies related to the blood vessels were found. One study aimed at simulating angiography (Luboz et al., 2013), and another aimed intravenous injection (Lee et al., 2012).

In the work for training of the angiography procedure, focused on an artery, two workstations were implemented. The workstation 1 was an AR environment and had a haptic device Geomagic Touch, mounted on the display frame at an angle of 45 degrees from vertical, the stereoscopic glasses to visualize the environment with virtual objects overlaid into the real scene, and a mannequin. The mannequin was composed by bony structure (e.g., anterior superior iliac spine, the pubic tubercle) made of hard plastic, muscle, and fat layer built with flexible expanded foam, skin made of silicone gel, and a pulse simulation block, connected to a system to feel a programmed pulse. The workstation 2 had silicon skin with an incision local to simulate the needle inserted in the artery and two specific electromechanical haptic devices, different from the other studies that used commercial devices. In this workstation, one device simulated the catheter, another simulated the needle, with a holder device that consisted of two frames to provide an axis of rotation along their servomotors and pressure position sensor (Luboz et al., 2013).

The user assessment was made in three steps (Luboz et al., 2013):

1. Ten experts, during a UK meeting of expert vascular interventional radiologists, analyzed the force feedback realism for the different anatomical structures simulated.
2. Fifty-two people, in six UK hospitals, participated in the experiment, to specify the relevance of measures, incorporated in the simulator, in terms of acceptability, performance assessment, and the effectiveness of the simulator in the training. Similar to the work of Chowriappa et al. (2015), the study was conducted in more than one hospital.
3. Sixty-four participants, with different levels of expertise in interventional radiology, split into two groups: group 1 consisted of participants with 0 to 4 years experience (41 participants), and group 2 consisted of participants with 5 or more years of experience (23 participants). The beginners were in the group 1, according to the years of experience in the area of interest. The measures analyzed were: needle passes through skin (count), needle passes through artery (count), distance between anaesthetic and puncture (mm), number of no go areas hit (count), times taken on workstation 1 and workstation 2.

In the work for training of the intravenous injection procedure, similar to previous study presented, focused also in a blood vessel as target body region and used a specific electromechanical haptic device. The system had a monitor, a webcam, a silicon leg in a fur skin, and the haptic device: a syringe with gyrosensors and force feedback generators, attached a button and Light-Emitting Diode (LED) markers (Lee et al., 2012).

The user evaluation was with 60 beginners, considering certain bases, such as fixing a leg, finding the vein, injection, and overall success. This is the only study related to veterinary education. Another issue about this research, the audio was implemented in this AR system (Lee et al., 2012).

There are studies with AR systems that did not employ electromechanical devices (specific or commercial equipment). These works used real artificial objects to provide haptic sensations, supporting sensors to capture data that were transferred to the computer to the simulation of the training.

One work, published in the year 2014, aimed at simulating the training of the vertebroplasty or kyphoplasty procedure. The target body region is the spine, similar to various studies cited. The system had the following parts: mannequin (torso), monitor, tracking system, and medical instruments usually handled in this type of procedure. Artificial skin and vertebrae were built using silicone rubber and plastic, respectively (Fuerst et al., 2014).

User tests were not the objective of this work. The tests focused on the artificial real objects, analyzing the vertebrae. These artificial vertebrae were analyzed considering the format and stiffness, and comparison between artificial and human vertebrae. A device was used to capture information about stiffness when the needle reaches a structure (Fuerst et al., 2014).

There is a study that did not address a specific procedure, developing a system composed of a mannequin (abdomen) on the table, a projector, fiducial markers in the wall and table, an optical tracking system based on infrared (fusionTrack 500, Atracsys LLC, Switzerland), and a needle applicator tracked by identifying optical markers (Heinrich et al., 2019a).

The user evaluation was conducted with 25 participants. Subjective and objective tests were also applied, using a questionnaire for analyzing the difficulties of the users; and certain measures, such as positioning, orientation and depth of the needle during the insertion to determine the accuracy (Heinrich et al., 2019a).

The same research group that made the previous study, worked in an AR-based system for training in spinal intervention. This system is composed of: marker, mannequin, a needle applicator, and HoloLens, an optical see-through HMD developed by Microsoft (Heinrich et al., 2019b).

The user evaluation was conducted with 21 beginners. An apparatus was also created for comparison with the system. The apparatus consisted of: a registration board, a floral foam bricks, a needle applicator, a HoloLens, and a control pad. Subjective and objective assessments were made, in which for each training session, the measure used was the task completion time, measured between the beginning of the insertion process and when the needle was pulled out of the target. After the participation, beginners were asked how level (easy or difficult) to find the correct insertion angle (subjective task difficulty) and how confident they were to have inserted the needle correctly (accuracy confidence) (Heinrich et al., 2019b).

Finally, the last study described also had the spine as the target body region, in a spinal anesthesia procedure. Four beginners and one expert participated in the user evaluation, and the researchers applied NASA-TLX (cognitive assessment) and used measures, such as procedure time, success, and normalized needle path-length (Ameri et al., 2019). Again, subjective and objective tests are made in the user assessment.

The system has an artificial real object, 3D printed, to represent a spine, that was fixed in a box, and in this box a tracking sensor was attached. Additionally, the system uses a mixture of gelatin and metamucil fiber model soft tissue, and a mixture of gelatin and barium sulfate to simulate the dura and ligamentum flavum.

The model of the epidural space uses gelatin without any scattering agents (Ameri et al., 2019).

8.5 ANALYSIS OF THE STUDIES

In this section, the studies described in the previous section were analyzed, according to characteristics extracted from articles, such as publications per year, medical procedure, target body region, devices (electromechanical or based on artificial real objects, commercial or specific), user assessment (measures, numbers of participants, beginners, and experts).

Regarding the publications per year, Figure 8.2 shows the chart with the number of studies per year found in the literature, between 2011 and 2019, and that are relevant contributions to science.

Two research groups published four studies (two works for each group), in the years 2011 and 2019. In the years 2016, 2017, and 2018 there were no publications. Thus, each year one or two works were published about AR-based systems with haptic devices for needle insertion training.

Regarding the procedure and target body region, one study did not specify a procedure and a target body region (Heinrich et al., 2019a). The authors analyzed concepts to simulate the needle insertion task with the projection of virtual information in the real world, superimposed in an artificial patient. Figure 8.3 shows the medical procedures identified and Figure 8.4 shows the target body regions. Both present the number of studies for each procedure and target body region.

Vertebroplasty is a type of spinal intervention and both were grouped (Heinrich et al., 2019b; Fuerst et al., 2014; Sutherland et al., 2011, 2013). Two studies that focused on spinal intervention were of the same research group (Sutherland et al., 2011, 2013). It is possible to observe that there are different procedures, except spinal intervention.

Analyzing the target body regions, the spine is the predominant region (Ameri et al., 2019; Heinrich et al., 2019b; Sutherland et al., 2011, 2013). Artery (Luboz et al., 2013; Coles et al., 2011b) and blood vessel regions (Lee et al., 2012) were grouped.

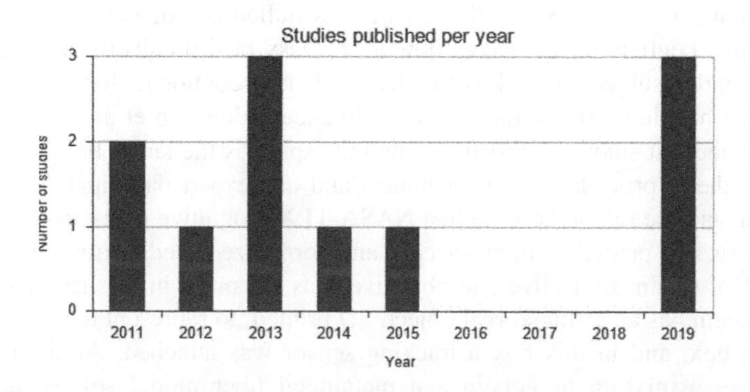

FIGURE 8.2 Number of Studies Analyzed According to the Publication Year.

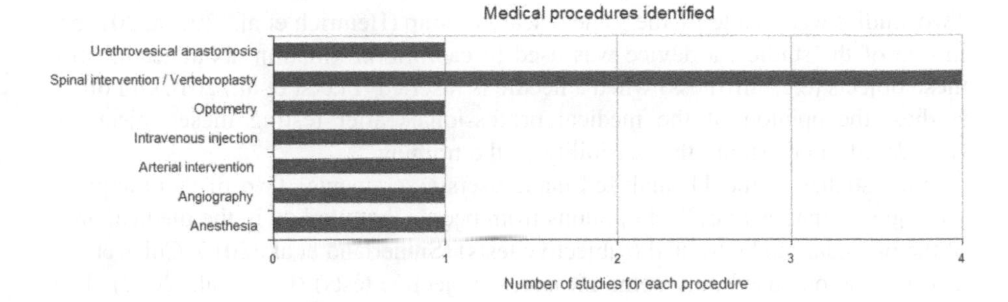

FIGURE 8.3 Number of Studies for Each Procedure Identified in Which Needle Insertion Is a Relevant Task.

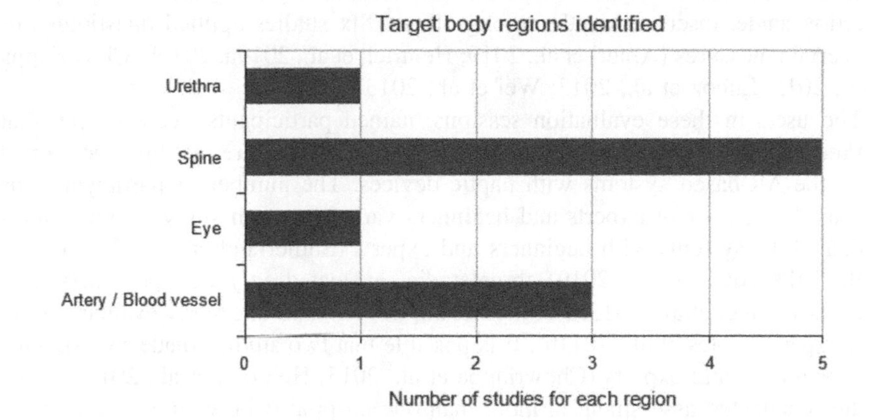

FIGURE 8.4 Number of Studies for Each Target Body Region Identified in Which Needle Insertion Is an Important Task.

Regarding the haptic devices, nine electromechanical haptic devices were found: three specific devices (Luboz et al., 2013, Lee et al., 2012) and six commercial electromechanical devices (Chowriappa et al., 2015; Luboz et al., 2013; Wei et al., 2013; Sutherland et al., 2011, 2013; Coles et al., 2011a,b,c). Of these commercial devices, there are three Geomagic Touch (Luboz et al., 2013; Wei et al., 2013; Coles et al., 2011a,b,c), two Phantom Premium 1.5 (Sutherland et al., 2011, 2013) and one robot for having surgery (daVinci Surgical System) (Chowriappa et al., 2015). The Geomagic Touch device was modified, removing the stylus and connecting a real needle hub. Phantom Premium 1.5 device was the same, used in two studies analyzed; and two specific devices were presented in the same article (Luboz et al., 2013). Two Novint Falcon devices were used in a research, but to simulate the palpation task, while Geomagic Touch simulated the needle insertion task (Coles et al., 2011b).

In addition to electromechanical haptic devices, four artificial real objects with sensors for providing touch, especially objects that represent anatomical structures, were built (Heinrich et al., 2019a, 2019b; Ameri et al., 2019; Fuerst et al., 2014).

Two studies were made by the same research group (Heinrich et al., 2019a, 2019b). In one of the studies, a device was used to capture information about features of these objects (e.g., stiffness) when a needle is inserted (Fuerst et al., 2014). In other studies, the opinion of the medical professionals after testing these objects is considered to determine the feasibility in the training.

Nine studies of the 11 analyzed made users assessments. Two of them applied only questionnaires to collect opinions from people that worked in the medical area of the procedure to be trained (subjective tests) (Sutherland et al., 2013; Coles et al., 2011b); and one used only some measures (objective tests) (Lee et al., 2012). The questionnaires have items to check ease of use, satisfaction of the user, realism provided by the system, among others. The measures employed, that deal with aspects of the needle insertion task, were: time taken to complete the task, the number of contacts with structures that were not the target region, insertion point, insertion angle, insertion depth, among others. Six studies applied questionnaires and certain measures (Ameri et al., 2019; Heinrich et al., 2019a, 2019b; Chowriappa et al., 2015; Luboz et al., 2013; Wei et al., 2013).

The users in these evaluation sessions, named participants, were people that worked (experts) and will work (beginners) with the procedure that must be trained using the AR-based systems with haptic devices. The number of participants, as well as the number of experts and beginners varied for each study. Three studies evaluated the systems with beginners and experts (Sutherland et al., 2013; Luboz et al., 2013; Ameri et al., 2019), three studies evaluated only with beginners (Lee et al., 2012; Wei et al., 2013; Heinrich et al., 2019b), and one study evaluated only with experts (Coles et al., 2011b). It is possible that two studies made experiments with beginners and experts (Chowriappa et al., 2015; Heinrich et al., 2019a). Two studies conducted assessment in more than one hospital (Chowriappa et al., 2015; Luboz et al., 2013).

In four studies, the number of participants for each evaluation was equal to or less than 10. In the works with experts and beginners, the number of beginners was usually greater than experts. It is important to mention that assessment with human beings has research projects submitted to an Ethical Committee to be appreciated, ensuring the safety of the participants.

It is possible to observe that there is not a standard evaluation protocol, varying the types of questionnaires and measures, number of participants (beginners and experts), because there are different procedures, although the main task is needle insertion.

Haptic feedback was combined with graphical effects in most of the works. Sound effects were implemented in one system, that was the only for veterinary education (Lee et al., 2012). Common video monitors were used in several simulators; HMD, stereoscopic glasses, and projectors were underexplored.

8.6 CHALLENGES, TRENDS, AND OPPORTUNITIES

Among the identified trends, needle insertion medical training using AR systems and haptic devices involves the wide use of commercial electromechanical haptic devices. Besides, 3D printers can be useful in building physical objects to representing anatomical structures (e.g., bones), in which projective AR systems can superimpose virtual tissues on these physical structures.

Another trend is the wide use of the Geomagic Touch device, because of the cost and benefit for the needle insertion task. As a customization, it is possible to replace the stylus with a medical instrument used in the medical procedure, such as a needle holder or a syringe. We concluded the cost is a relevant factor for the device to be integrated with the systems.

Our review of the literature presented a great exploration of visual and haptic feedback combined. However, among the challenges and opportunities we found, sound feedback was under-explored. Additionally, none of the systems analyzed implemented gamification techniques that aim at adding game elements (e.g., scores, ranking, and awards).

In the past years, tools for developing AR systems have been improved, including systems for smartphones and tablets, such as ARKit (Apple Inc., 2020) and ARCore (Google Developers, 2020). These software development kits offer resources for virtual objects rendering and real environment tracking. The tracking can be made without markers, using features of the real environment.

With the use of smart see-through glasses and smartphone, Li et al. (2019) developed an AR system that can provide needle guidance for transperineal prostate procedure. Using Unity and Vuforia SDK platforms, Hecht et al. (2020) developed an AR smartphone application for needle insertion guidance with potential to improve needle insertion accuracy.

Pseudo-haptic approaches are not explored in the AR-based systems. The pseudo-haptic interaction aims at simulating haptic effects, such as stiffness, without the physical presence of an electromechanical haptic device. These effects are created using visual changes in graphical interfaces according to touch or gestures (Lécuyer et al., 2000). Thus, pseudo-haptic can be used in smartphones with touch screens, allowing the use of mobile devices and preventing equipment with robotic arms attached.

A problem identified in AR systems for needle insertion medical training is the limitation imposed by the shape of the part handled by the user in the haptic device. As these devices are of general use, the representation of the simulated needle does not have the same shape as the equivalent real object. Although some approaches replace these parts of the haptic device with needles or syringes, it would be more appropriate for the manufacturer of these devices to design them to be modularized, with replaceable parts as needed for the application. In this way, AR systems based on such devices could offer participants an experience closer to the real one. The constant use of haptic devices in medical training, in general, may indicate to the manufacturers of these devices the need for specific or adaptable equipment for a particular type of training. Needle insertion training is an example of such an application.

When a VR system is used for medical training, the real environment is completely hidden by the virtual. This feature naturally does not allow the participant to view the haptic device in the scene regardless of the direction of the participant's gaze. In an AR system, parts of the real environment that are not overlapped by virtual elements are displayed to participants. Thus, in applications that simulate a needle insertion procedure, even if a virtual needle overlaps the part of the haptic device handled by the participant, the other parts of the equipment will be viewed. To achieve high levels of realism, it is important that systems hide parts of the haptic device that are not part of the training environment from the participant (e.g., the work of Coles et al., 2011b).

The purpose of AR systems that use haptic devices for needle insertion training is to simulate the application environment, including tactile and force feedback. Certain haptic devices, although they make it possible to generate systems with such resources, may not be suitable for use in this type of application for ergonomic reasons. A major challenge for manufacturers is to develop haptic devices that do not limit the movements of the participants needed to perform the procedure. It is thought that, for certain types of medical training, the challenge of producing suitable devices is practically insurmountable. However, specifically for needle insertion training, the evolution of the equipment currently found on the market indicates that some ergonomic limitations can be overcome in the short or medium term.

In addition to the improvements related to the devices, it is important that the software used follows the evolution of the equipment. The evolution of the software must occur in such a way that the full capacity of the haptic device is exploited. Another important aspect related to the software refers to its usability. The studies analyzed showed that the application of usability tests is frequent in medical training systems. Many of these tests even recruit users from the specific medical field in which the procedure under study is related and use different questionnaires and measures in the evaluation.

In addition to usability, it is desirable that AR systems that simulate needle insertion are robust so that the realism of the experience is not compromised due to software failures. An important step in the development process is the application of formal software testing methods, checking failures, as well as the faults in the source code that caused these failures. In the AR applications aimed at training needle insertion analyzed in this research, there is no report of tests performed in the simulator software. The performance of these tests is important because it directly influences the quality and reliability of the system.

The use of robots to mediate medical procedures may require other skills, which must be trained. The robots can be used in procedures that require precision in the medical instruments manipulation or in remote procedures.

8.7 CONCLUSION

There are various tools for procedures training in the medical area that use computers. The procedures usually involve the accurate manipulation of certain instruments, and knowledge and sensorimotor skills to carry out them, preventing injuries to the patients are fundamental to the success.

A task that is present in several medical procedures and must be trained is the needle insertion. Some procedures the medical professional performs with the support of images, and in certain cases, a sequence of images, from computed tomography, ultrasound, requiring manual skill while observing the anatomical structures and the needle in a monitor. Usually, the professional must manipulate the needle and a probe, which captures these images in real time. Other procedures consist of palpation and needle insertion tasks, which must be performed simultaneously. Finally, in others where there is no visual support, knowledge of anatomy and tactile sensation are the forms of professional guidance.

AR techniques (a blend of virtual and real elements in a 3D space) and haptic devices (to capture movements of the needle and provide touch sensations when the needle is inserted in anatomical structures) are useful in the development of training systems. In the literature, there are studies related to activities of development and assessment of systems, validating especially with users from medical areas.

This chapter presented some research challenges and opportunities in simulation-based needle insertion training. Besides, it showed that this technology is a trend in medical training, for offering the possibility of reducing training costs and risks inherent to the medical procedures.

REFERENCES

Aboud, E.; Suarez, C.; Al-Mefty, O.; Yasargil, M. New alternative to animal models for surgical training. Alternatives to Laboratory Animals 2004;32(Suppl 1B):S501–507.

Akhtar, K. S. N.; Chen, A.; Standfield, N. J.; Gupte, C. M. The role of simulation in developing surgical skills. Current Reviews in Musculoskeletal Medicine 2014;7(2): 155–160.

Ameri, G.; Rankin, A.; Baxter, J.; Moore, J.; Ganapathy, S.; Peters, T.; Chen, E. Development and evaluation of an augmented reality ultrasound guidance system for spinal anesthesia: Preliminary results. Ultrasound in Medicine & Biology 2019:45. 10.1016/j.ultrasmedbio.2019.04.026.

Apple Inc. Introducing ARKit 3.5 Pro. 2020. Available in: https://developer.apple.com/augmented-reality/arkit/. Access at: 30 Apr 2020.

Azuma, R. A survey of augmented reality. Teleoperators and Virtual Environments 1997;6(4):355–385.

Azuma, R. Overview of augmented reality. In: SIGGRAPH '04: ACM SIGGRAPH 2004 Course Notes. ACM Press, p. 26. 2004.

Balcombe, J. Medical training using simulation: Toward fewer animals and safer patients. Alternatives to Laboratory Animals 2004;32(Suppl 1B):S553–560.

Botden, S. M.; Jakimowicz, J. J. What is going on in augmented reality simulation in laparoscopic surgery? Surgical Endoscopy 2009;23(8):1693–1700.

Chaballout, Basil; Molloy, Margory; Vaughn, Jacqueline; Brisson, Raymond; Shaw, Ryan. Feasibility of augmented reality in clinical simulations: Using Google Glass with Manikins. JMIR Medical Education 2016;2(1):e2.

Chowriappa, A.; Raza, S.; Fazili, A.; Field, E.; Malito, C.; Samarasekera, D.; Shi, Y.; Ahmed, K.; Wilding, G.; Kaouk, J.; Eun, D. D.; Ghazi, A.; Peabody, J. O.; Kesavadas, T.; Mohler, J. L.; Guru, K. A. Augmented-reality-based skills training for robot-assisted urethrovesical anastomosis: A multi-institutional randomised controlled trial. BJU International 2015;115(2):336–345.

Coles, T. R.; John, N. W.; Gould, D. A.; Caldwell, D. G. Integrating haptics with augmented reality in a femoral palpation and needle insertion training simulation. IEEE Transactions on Haptics 2011b;4(3):199–209.

Coles, T. R.; John, N. W.; Sofia, G.; Gould, D. A.; Caldwell, D. G. Modification of commercial force feedback hardware for needle insertion simulation. Studies in Health Technology and Informatics 2011c;163:135–137.

Coles, T. R.; Meglan, D.; John, N. W. The role of haptics in medical training simulators: A survey of the state of the art. IEEE Transactions on Haptics 2011a; 4(1):51–66.

Corrêa, C. G.; Machado, M. A. A. M.; Ranzini, E.; Tori, R.; Nunes, F. L. S. Virtual Reality simulator for dental anesthesia training in the inferior alveolar nerve block. Journal of Applied Oral Science 2017;25(4).

Corrêa, C. G.; Nunes, F. L. S.; Ranzini, E.; Nakamura, R.; Tori, R. Haptic interaction for needle insertion training in medical applications: The state-of-the-art. Medical Engineering & Physics 2019;63:6–25. ISSN 1350-4533. 10.1016/j.medengphy.2018.11.002.

Eck, U.; Pankratz, F.; Sandor, C.; Klinker, G.; Laga, H. Precise haptic device co-location for visuo-haptic augmented reality. IEEE Transactions on Visualization and Computer Graphics 2015;21(12):1427–1441.

Fuerst, D.; Hollensteiner, M.; Schrempf, A. A novel augmented reality simulator for minimally invasive spine surgery. In: Proceedings of the Summer Simulation Multiconference (SummerSim'14) 2014;28:1–28.

Gomoll, A. H.; O'Toole, R. V.; Czarnecki, J.; Warner, J. J. P. Surgical experience correlates with performance on a virtual reality simulator for shoulder arthroscopy. American Journal of Sports Medicine 2007;35(6):883–888.

Google Developers. ARCore. 2020. Available in: <https://developers.google.com/ar>. Access at: 30 Apr 2020.

Grechenig, W.; Fellinger, M.; Fankhauser, F.; Weiglein, A. H. The graz learning and training model for arthroscopic surgery. Surgical and Radiologic Anatomy 1999;21(5):347–350.

Hassanien, A. E.; Dey, N.; Borra, S. (Eds.). Medical big data and internet of medical things: Advances, challenges and applications. CRC Press. 2018.

Hecht, R.; Li, M.; de Ruiter, Q. M. B.; Pritchard, W. F.; Li, X.; Krishnasamy, V.; Saad, W.; Karanian, J. W.; Wood, B. J. Smartphone augmented reality CT-based platform for needle insertion guidance: A phantom study. CardioVascular and Interventional Radiology 2020;43(5):756–764. 10.1007/s00270-019-02403-6.

Heinrich, F.; Joeres, F.; Lawonn, K.; Hansen, C. Comparison of projective augmented reality concepts to support medical needle insertion. IEEE Transactions on Visualization and Computer Graphics 2019a;25(6):2157–2167.

Heinrich, F.; Schwenderling, L.; Becker, M.; Skalej, M.; Hansen, C. HoloInjection: Augmented reality support for CT-guided spinal needle injections. Healthcare Technology Letters 2019b;6(6):165–171, 12.

Iacobucci, G. NHS wastes at least £1bn a year on avoidable errors, claims health secretary. BMJ 2014;349(October):g6287. 10.1136/bmj.g6287.

Jarillo-Silva, A.; Domínguez-Ramírez, O.; Parra-Vega, V.; Ordaz, P. PHANToM OMNI haptic device: kinematic and manipulability. In Electronics, Robotics and Automotive Mechanics Conference (CERMA) 2009, pp. 193–198.

Jaung, R.; Cook, P.; Blyth, P. A comparison of embalming fluids for use in surgical workshops. Clinical Anatomy 2011;24(2):155–161.

Lambden, S.; Martin B. The use of computers for perioperative simulation in anesthesia, critical care, and pain medicine. Anesthesiology Clinics 2011;29(3):521–531.

Lécuyer, A.; Coquillart, S.; Kheddar, A.; Richard, P.; Coiffet, P. Pseudo-haptic feedback: can isometric input devices simulate force feedback? IEEE Virtual Reality 2000:83–90.

Lee, J.; Kim, W.; Seo, A.; Jun, J.; Lee, S.; Kim, J.-I.; Eom, K.; Pyeon, M.; Lee, H. An intravenous injection simulator using augmented reality for veterinary education and its evaluation. In: Proceedings of the Eleventh ACM SIGGRAPH International

Conference on Virtual-Reality Continuum and Its Applications in Industry (VRCAI'12) 2012:31–34.

Li, M.; Xu, S.; Mazilu, D.; Turkbey, B.; Wood, B. J. Smartglasses/smartphone needle guidance AR system for transperineal prostate procedures. In Medical Imaging 2019: Image-guided Procedures, Robotic Interventions, and Modeling. International Society for Optics and Photonics, Vol. 10951, p. 109510Z. 2019.

Luboz, V.; Zhang, Y.; Johnson, S.; Song, Y.; Kilkenny, C.; Hunt, C.; Woolnough, H.; Guediri, S.; Zhai, J.; Odetoyinbo, T.; Littler, P.; Fisher, A.; Hughes, C.; Chalmers, N.; Kessel, D.; Clough, P. J.; Ward, J.; Phillips, R.; How, T.; Bulpitt, A.; John, N. W.; Bello, F.; Gould, D. Imagine seldinger: First simulator for seldinger technique and angiography training. Computer Methods and Programs in Biomedicine 2013;111(2):419–434.

Makary, M. A.; Daniel, M. Medical error – the third leading cause of death in the us. BMJ 2016:353.

O'Neill, M. J.; Milano, M. T.; Schell, M. C. Simulation training in health care: A role in radiation oncology? International Journal of Radiation Oncology, Biology, Physics 2011;81(2):697–698.

Salisbury, K.; Conti, F.; Barbagli, F. Haptic rendering: Introductory concepts. IEEE Computer Graphics and Applications 2004;24(2):24–32.

Shakil, O.; Mahmood, F.; Matyal, R. Simulation in echocardiography: An ever-expanding frontier. Journal of Cardiothoracic and Vascular Anesthesia 2012;26(3):476–485.

Shinde, G. R.; Dhotre, P. S.; Mahalle, P. N.; Dey, N. Internet of things integrated augmented reality. Springer, Singapore. 2020.

Sutherland, C.; Hashtrudi-Zaad, K.; Abolmaesumi, P.; Mousavi, P. Towards an augmented ultrasound guided spinal needle insertion system. In: Proceedings of the Annual International Conference of the IEEE Engineering in Medicine and Biology Society (EMBC'11) 2011:3459–3462.

Sutherland, C.; Hashtrudi-Zaad, K.; Sellens, R.; Abolmaesumi, P.; Mousavi, P. An augmented reality haptic training simulator for spinal needle procedures. IEEE Transactions on Biomedical Engineering 2013;60(11):3009–3018.

Tang, K.; Cheng, D.; Mi, E.; Greenberg, P. Augmented reality in medical education: A systematic review. Canadian Medical Education Journal 2020;11:e81–e96. 10.36834/cmej.61705.

Ullrich, S.; Kuhlen, T. Haptic palpation for medical simulation in virtual environments. IEEE Transactions on Visualization and Computer Graphics 2012;18(4):617–625. 10.1109/TVCG.2012.46.

Vadalà, G.; Salvatore, S. D.; Ambrosio, L.; Russo, F.; Papalia, R.; Denaro, V. Robotic spine surgery and augmented reality systems: A state of the art. Neurospine 2020;17(1):88–100.

Varalakshmi, B. D.; Thriveni, J; Venugopal, K. R.; Patnaik, L. M. Haptics: State of the art survey. International Journal of Computer Science Issues (IJCSI) 2012;9(5):234–244.

Wang, X.; Dunston, P. S. Design, strategies, and issues towards an augmented reality-based construction training platform. ITcon 2007;12:363–380.

Wei, L.; Nahavandi, S.; Weisinger H. Optometry training simulation with augmented reality and haptics. In: Proceedings of the 2013 IEEE/ACM International Conference on Advances in Social Networks Analysis and Mining (ASONAM'13) 2013:976–977.

Willis, R. E.; Gomez, P. P.; Ivatury, S. J.; Mitra, H. S.; Sickle, K. R.V. Virtual reality simulators: Valuable surgical skills trainers or video games? Journal of Surgical Education 2014;71(3):426–433.

9 Current Strategies and Future Perspectives of Autoimmune Disorder

Satya Narayan Sahu[1], Biswajit Mishra[1], Rojalin Sahu[1], and Subrat Kumar Pattanayak[2]

[1]School of Applied Sciences, Kalinga Institute of Industrial Technology (KIIT), Deemed to be University, Bhubaneswar, India

[2]Department of Chemistry, National Institute of Technology, Raipur, India

CONTENTS

9.1 INTRODUCTION: BACKGROUND AND DRIVING FORCES

Digital technology or computer technology plays an important role in the modern healthcare system, such as clinical diagnosis, treatment, medical imaging, and medical data management and analysis [1]. Now, the use of digital technology in modeling, analyzing, formulating, and solving problems in medicine is very crucial [2]. Information technology/electronic communication or computational technology is the union of digital technologies such as digital information, communication, and data to share, collect, and analyze the health information to improve health care system and health. Both hardware and software solutions are used in digital healthcare technology. By adopting this technology, healthcare professionals can manage their patients with different illnesses and health risks [3]. This digital healthcare system includes monitoring and assessment to treat, prevent, and diagnose different types of diseases. It includes analysis and optimal segmentation in 3D images like blood clots, vascular network, airways, joint structures, motion tracking of bacteria in 3D image movies, etc. [4]. It is a multidisciplinary area which involves researchers, scientists, and clinicians having a broad range of expertise in different disciplines like engineering, chemistry, informatics, healthcare, public

DOI: 10.1201/9781003198796-9

health, social science, government sector hospitals, professional organizations, various regulatory bodies, industries, economics, etc. [5,6]. The most important contribution of computational healthcare system is to minimize the cost without compromising the healthcare services [7,8]. It also has the prospective to stimulate, optimize, and streamline the clinical research. It can also be used to monitor patients for rehabilitation or long-term care. It also helps people with any kind of disabilities with everyday work by the help of assistive technologies or robotics. Cochlear implants [9] are offered to patients with hearing and speech disorders. Telemedicine, telecare, telehealth, and tele-rehabiliation are supplied to patients in remote areas. People are unable to meet the needs of their complex diseases because of the limited resources of the healthcare system in rural areas [10]. The introduction of telehealth care or the Internet of Things (IoT)-based healthcare system will resolve the concerns and needs of people with disabilities living in rural areas. In order to meet the specialist doctors to get better care and to evaluate and interpret patient-related data, computer-based systems, such as the Clinical Decision Support System, are also used. Machine learning and modeling of simulations will help healthcare systems [11,12].

Further, E-health provides information on health and many services to facilitate data storage, data transmission, and recovery for different uses in clinical, administrative, and educational purposes [13]. These technologies facilitate and also are much more conventional for clinical trials. Nowadays, mobile computing adds value to clinicians in different ways like information exchange, reducing errors due to inadequate availability of clinical information, and helps in making clinical decisions at point of care. Digital healthcare is now enriched with the data generated by various medical devices. Sometimes, this massive data remain unused, may be due to the lack of analysts or scientists [14]. This is the reason for which it is not able to meet the demand of the continuously growing big data. Big data is well known for its wide application in healthcare sector for management of data [15]. There are some reports regarding the big data and IoT, which are extremely important for future healthcare system with an affordable cost.

The abundant data related to health collected from various resources like medical imaging, pharmaceutical research, biomedical research, medical devices, electronic health records, etc. are known as big data. The data is generated from various sources and its volume is too high as well as it is extremely variable in its structure and nature. Big data needs appropriate management and analysis to derive useful information from it. High-end computing solutions as well as appropriate infrastructures are required in healthcare sectors to overcome various challenges in analysis of big data [16]. Efficient management, interpretation, and analysis of this huge data can help healthcare sector immensely. Presently, all the healthcare industries are taking strong steps for converting the data from big data base for the betterment of healthcare and to make healthcare services more economical. Integrating healthcare and data generated from biomedical research may bring a revolution in personalized medicine and therapies. As a prototype, big data is being used to process data for the latest Internet revolution, i.e., IoT, which has a very important role in the area of healthcare.

IoT is really an evolution in the healthcare system and before IoT, interaction of patients with doctors or healthcare professionals, recommendation of particular treatments limiting the visit of patients to hospitals and clinics. It is immensely helpful for disabled patients, elderly patients, and patients residing in remote areas, keeping them safe as well as healthy. Further, it empowers doctors to deliver best healthcare, increasing satisfaction and involvement of patients.

The most important benefits of IoT in healthcare system are:

- **Economical treatment by reducing cost**: Real-time monitoring of health of patients considerably reduces the cost because it avoids admission, visit to the hospital or health clinics, and therefore eliminates the bed charges and other charges during the stay in the hospital.
- **Advanced treatment to the patients**: IoT facilitates evidence-based transparent decisions for the patients.
- **Early diagnosis of the disease**: Constant and real-time monitoring of patients helps in the early stage diagnosis of diseases on the basis of symptoms.
- **Dynamic treatment**: Constant monitoring of health of patients provides dynamic treatment to the patients in real sense.
- **Proper management of medical instruments and medicines**: The major challenge in healthcare system is medical instruments as well as drugs which can be managed very well by the help of IoT, reducing the treatment cost.
- **Treatment with minimal error**: The data gathered by IoT enable very smooth healthcare operation with minimal error.
- **Facilitation of patient care by IoT**: Patients can use smart devices such as fitness bands, blood pressure and heart rate monitors, glucometers, smartphone apps, etc. which give personalized healthcare. These smart devices can be tuned which, then, can remind the patients about their calorie intake, exercise, blood sugar level variations so that patient can decide if there is need for doctor visit or no. It will also help the patients in early diagnosis and keep the patient notified about any uncertain risk. It also reduces the stress and confusion of the patients.
- **Location of hospital by IoT-based smartphone app or smart badges**: IoT-based smartphone apps help patients find a hospital in a nearby location and sometimes it is used to send information to the hospitals about the location of the patient resulting in increased patient satisfaction. Sensor badges, worn by a patient, can track where his/her position in the process during operations and family members of the concerned patient can stay updated.
- **Facilitation of IoT for healthcare professionals**: Using smart devices, doctors can track the health of the patients and they can adhere to different treatment modalities or requirement of any medical attention. Hence, physicians can be much more connected to the patients and can be more watchful to their patients and can have the expected outcomes of the treatments.
- **Benefits from IoT to hospitals**: IoT-based devices can monitor hygiene in the hospital and help reduce infections in patients. Engagement of equipments and hospital staffs can also be monitored in real time. Assets like pharmacy, environment like humidity, temperature control of refrigerators by smart fridges, especially for fridges storing vaccines can monitor temperature

remotely, etc. can be controlled by IoT-based devices. Smart refrigerators also streamline the interaction process with vaccines allowing data analysis and storage of vaccines to be distributed in high risk remote areas.

- **Benefits from IoT to health insurance companies**: Flexibility and customization can be achieved by health insurance companies with the introduction of IoT. Data generated through IoT provides information about their product or services as well as advices and demonstrates the insured members about the care to be taken. The data generated by these intelligent devices can help in claims operations. These devices also help maintain transparency between insurers and costumers, which helps in decision-making in every outcome.

Basically, IoT comprises computing devices and digital and mechanical machines [17]. IoT has the capability of exchanging data in an intelligent way over the Internet without any interaction between humans or human and computer. The rapid communication occurs converging data, communication network, cloud, and devices. The setup comprises devices such as sensors, Internet TV, and appliances like thermostats, camera, light fixtures and other appliances, which can be controlled by devices like smartphones and smart speakers. IoT cannot help stop aging in population or eliminate deadly diseases but it can definitely make healthcare easier in terms of ease of accessibility. By using this technology, there will be improvements in the quality as well as efficiency in treatment of patients. IoT not only helps in making accessibility to healthcare easy but is also very helpful in research in this sector. IoT enables collecting a large amount of patient-related data which could be almost impossible in case of manual collection. This data can serve useful in statistical studies which can support the healthcare research. Here, we can say that this facility is not only saving time but also our money and is helping in medical research. For example, the IoT devices transfer patient's health-related data such as blood pressure, sugar levels in the blood, weight, and ECG, etc. which can be stored in cloud and can be shared privately with the concerned person, may be a doctor, insurance company, health consultant, etc. who can refer the data without the need for patient visit, thereby saving time. This makes the healthcare service more effective and deliverable. IoT can promote patient care and helps mobility of healthcare and new technologies as well as enables next-generation healthcare system. It also helps in machine-to-machine communication, exchange of information, and exchange of data, which will bring a great change in healthcare system. In this way, IoT enables doctors as well as other healthcare professionals to be much more attentive and connected to the patients.

IoT has been used in many devices that augment the quality of healthcare received by patients with many diseases. IoT helps in managing drugs, reducing the staff, waiting time for patients, and helping in making critical care available for patients. Several IoT-based devices have made patients lives more comfortable. Furthermore, IoT can manage personalize healthcare services with complete maintenance of identity for each and every individual. Many types of equipment are utilized in healthcare to communicate between the healthcare professionals and the patients. The IoT combines conventional domains including automation and control system, combination of hardware and software systems, which is collectively known as embedded system, wireless sensor networks for device-to-device through Internet. The primary requirement for IoT implementation is the Radio Frequency Identification (RFID). The IoT system offers a platform to identify and link physical surroundings to the virtual world through the global Internet. These objects may be medical equipments like sensors. The action on the physical objects and their resources can be restored by virtual manifestation. The typical way of healthcare is restricted by the time and availability of hospitals or clinics, i.e., a patient has to visit a doctor and has to wait in the waiting room. Sometimes, the patients residing in remote areas are not able to avail these facilities. Patients who are in their old age and handicapped patients face many difficulties in visiting the hospitals and clinics. The barriers can be effectively broken by a powerful tool, i.e., Information and Communication Technology (ICT). Conventional healthcare methods offer delayed services because of the location of hospitals and clinics as well as medical facilities. This can be developed with IoT services and by healthcare professionals and patients. A number of complex algorithms and sensors are used for analysis of data and then the analyzed data is shared through wireless medium to get recommendations from healthcare professionals remotely [18]. The clinical care monitors IoT system for hospitalization of patients. IoT system contains many systems for observations of patients.

Here, by using computational tools and software, we want to demonstrate some bioinformatics approaches to classify drug metabolisms and target-based drug interactions with biomolecules. This technique may be used to recognize a patient's preliminary drug response. We download the primary data from the cloud-based database for this operation. In this current research, we describe an example of autoimmune disorders in order to illustrate the process. Autoimmune disorders are caused due to overactive immune system [19]. These disorders cause damage to the body tissues and lead to abnormality in growth and function of various organs [20]. This disease may attack one or more organs in the body. The different parts of the body which are affected by these disorders are blood, skin, joints, and various cells [21]. There are various types of these diseases starting from rheumatoid, thyroid, type-1 diabetes, pulmonary fibrosis, etc. Immune system basically includes many parts of our body, such as some blood cells, bone marrow, skin, which helps keep us healthy [22]. This system protects us from varieties of infections. It fights against the infections by detecting infectious agents such as bacteria and viruses. This property of this system is called immune response of the body. The immune system attacks healthy cells instead of attacking the infectious agents, which leads to autoimmune disorders. The cause of the autoimmune diseases is not clearly understood. Autoimmune conditions affect the genetic susceptibility of developing a particular type of disease in the body [23]. This disorder is triggered by environmental factors like stress, diet, infection, and sometimes UV radiation. There are more than 80 types of these disorders.

9.2 AUTOIMMUNE DISORDERS

These diseases are basically associated with long-term sickness and become severe with time. Rheumatoid arthritis, an autoimmune disorder, occurs due to damage to the cartilage, which leads to stiffness and swollen in joints [24,25]. The disease, Lupus, affects various parts of the body starting from skin to heart. A disease of similar kind called celiac causes diarrhea, pain in the abdomen, and damage to the intestine [26,27]. Type-1 diabetes is also a similar disorder and it occurs due to insufficient secretion of insulin in pancreases of the patients [28,29]. Graves' disease is another commonly occurring autoimmune disease caused by overactive thyroid gland and causes anxiety, loss in weight, and irritation in eyes [30,31]. The main problem of this disease is its late diagnosis because symptoms take a longer time to feel the seriousness of the disease. There does not exist any medical test which can diagnose this kind of diseases. The large part of our income is dedicated to the treatment of this disease. It also contributes in a larger scale to morbidity and mortality. Every day, new cases are being reported and now it is increasing with an alarming rate. These diseases are chronic and millions of dollars are spent for the treatment and management of these disorders [32]. The disorder can be caused due to damage in the tissue or it may be systemic. However, all such disorders are due to an imbalance in the immune system in the body [33]. A healthy immune system recognizes and react to the pathogens [34]. Mainly, thymus lymphocytes or T cells have the capacity to respond to the foreign pathogens [35]. These cells are continuously generated in the thymus. Chemical-induced and auto-induced autoimmune diseases are basically affected by the T lymphocytes which is suggested by the study of animal models. Traditionally, these diseases are treated by immunosuppressive medications. These medications are very effective in case of many patients. But, long-term treatment of this disease with very high doses of the medicines sometimes causes the risk of malignancy. Therefore, the traditional drugs have less side effects as well as low toxicity. Hence, there is an urgency of strategies that will increase the tolerance. The main goal of the therapeutics is: (i) should be site specific, (ii) minimum toxicity, (iii) economical, and (iv) re-establishment of immune tolerance so that long-term treatment would not be required. The new advance treatment systems are struggling to achieve these goals. Most of the autoimmune disorders are caused due to overexpression of cytochrome P450 protein in various tissues in different organs.

Cytochrome P450 is the heme-containing protein [36]. It is termed as cytochrome P450 because the protein is a complex of porphyrin and iron as well as carbon monoxide and it absorbs at the wavelength of light (λmax) 450 nm. Here, the heme is bound noncovalently to the polypeptide chain of the proteins. During the metabolic process, this enzyme requires a molecule of oxygen and a water molecule and one oxidized product. In many cases depending on the nature of the substrate, it also requires more oxygen molecules than the metabolized substrates and sometimes produces oxides and superoxides. The heme group present in these systems is alkylated by the compounds formed from the acetylinic groups present in various substrates. This intermediate also binds to the protein in a covalent bond. Many biosynthetic and metabolic pathways are associated with these proteins or enzymes [37,38]. The significant role of this enzyme is in the metabolism of various therapeutic drugs and chemicals. These are also active in lipid metabolism. These enzymes also metabolize the fatty acids like omega-3 or omega-6. These are also very active in the synthesis of bile and cholesterol as well as vitamin A and vitamin D in the body. There are 57 types of Cytochrome P450 genes present in the human genome. These genes contain both active and pseudo genes. The function of

Cytochrome P450 is very important and, for example, mitochondiral Cytochrome P450 proteins are involved in the electrotransfer reaction that converts NADPH to Cytochrome P450. The most abundant Cytochrome P450 found in liver and intestine is Cytochrome P450 3A4 which metabolizes a number of endo- and exogenous compounds with diversified chemical structures. The expression of Cytochrome P450 3A sub family in human intestine is 70% and 30% of the total Cytochrome P450 is present in the liver tissues of human beings. These proteins are very important in the breakdown of almost all therapeutic drugs. These proteins are stabilized by different substrates and are highly unstable in case of oxidative stress. From literature, it is known that the arachidonic acid is metabolized by this family of Cytochrome P450 into 20 different hydroxyeicosatetraenoic (20-HETE) acids. These acids breakdown into substrates that affect the renal peripheral and tubular transport. This new acid which is generated due to the catalysis is very potent in stopping the sodium transport in proximal tubule. These are also altering the development of hypertension and renal injury which is confirmed by the preclinical studies. Normally, a foreign compound undergoes metabolism by a group of enzymes as soon an as it enters to the human body [39]. These enzymes which are actively associated with the metabolic processes are called xenobiotic-metabolizing enzymes. These enzymes are not only catalyzing in eukaryotic cells but also in prokaryotic cells. The most important xenobiotic-metabolizing enzymes are Cytochrome P450, which is embedded in the bilayers of phospholipids of endoplasmic reticulum. Many human Cytochrome P450 enzymes exhibit polymorphism [40]. Toxic quinones are generated by the catalytic conversion of various xenobiotics. Superoxide is generated due to interaction of redox sensitive agents with these quinones. It interacts with almost all type of drugs which is the primary aim to study its mechanism of interactions. The other unique properties associated with this family are its autoactivation by different substrates and its stimulation by flavonoids. The protein is induced by a number of drugs like phenobarbital and glucocortoids. It also plays a vital role in the metabolism of immunosuppressive drugs such as cyclosporine, antibiotics, namely erythromycin. These enzymes catalyze a variety of steroids such as progesterone, cortisol, testosterone, etc. This protein is used as an evaluator of the metabolism of erythromycin metabolism by testing the breath [41]. Recombinant of this protein is found in small organisms like *E. coli*, yeasts, and many cell lines. The recombinant Cytochrome P450 3A4 is involved in the metabolism of substrates like testosterone, nifedipene, lidocaine, etc. In case of humans, these proteins are expressed in lymphoblastoid cells [42,43]. These proteins are used to study the mutagenic as well as cytotoxic response to various drugs. Metabolism of xenobiotics by Cytochrome P450 produces Reactive Oxygen Species (ROS) and this ROS is very important for autoimmune response. This protein is also important in the pathology of various types of autoimmune disorders [44,45]. Some of these proteins are involved in the detoxication of xenobiotics. The reactive intermediates produced during the catalysis process can damage the DNA and also can be harmful for lipids and proteins. Chand et al. [46] studied the antiaging-related phytochemicals like curcumin, quercetin, and resveratrol with cytochrome P450 3A4 protein by molecular docking method and summarized that both hydrophobic as well as hydrogen bonding actively plays an important role in the interaction of these phytochemicals and Cytochrome P450 3A4 protein. Balasubramanian and coworkers [47] identified the components of the *Ocimum sanctum* leaf extract through gas chromatography–mass spectroscopy. Baliga et al. [48] studied the phytochemicals of tulsi plant with cancer preventative and its radioprotective properties.

Thus, by using various bioinformatics approaches through different computational methods and software, we strive to predict the drug binding site or target site of drugs. The binding sites, drug activity, and drug reaction to the protein cytochrome P450 3A4 are predicted by this current strategy. In order to predict the binding efficiency of the three-dimensional structure of the cytochrome P450 3A4 protein and various phytocompounds such as cyclohexane, 1,2,4-triethenyl- [47], apigenin [48], eugenol [48], we used the AutoDock toolkit for this analysis.

9.3 PROTOCOL USED DURING DOCKING PROCESS

The three-dimensional structure of cytochrome P450 3A4 was retrieved from the protein data bank (PDB) database having PDB Id 5VVC. The three-dimensional structure of studied protein have many splits within the structure, so for the interaction study we rebuild or construct the split by using discovery studio visualizing software. The resolution of cytochrome P450 3A4 crystal structure is 1.74 Å. The three-dimensional structure of studied protein structure was proceeded for analyzing the drug binding site with different phytochemical compounds and binding confirmations of the protein by using AutoDock Vina 4.2 [49] and the process is called molecular docking. The molecular docking is a computational process to find the binding performance between two small molecules. The small molecules are protein-drug or two chemical compounds. In the docking process, out of two molecules one is taken as a receptor and the other is considered a ligand, in which we have to make a grid box on receptor. In the present study, the three-dimensional structure of cytochrome p450 3A4 protein was taken as receptor and different phytochemicals like cyclohexane, 1,2,4-triethenyl- [47], apigenin [48], and eugenol [48] are considered as ligand. After removal of all the bad contacts from the receptor and ligand we calculated the Kollman charges and added the hydrogen atoms to the polar contacts of the receptor by using AutoDockTool-1.5.6. During the docking the AutoDock tool uses gradient optimization algorithm to perform the process. For the present studied receptor we calculated the grid box size of 98 × 98 × 98 in x, y, and z direction and center_x, center_y, and center_z are -21.767, -24.329, and -7.193, respectively. The structure preparation and visualization are of made by using Pymol visualizer software [50] and discovery studio visualizer software [51]. Followed by the interaction study we proceed for the computational drug likeness test for the studied phytochemicals by using SwissADME server [52], which is managed by Swiss Institute of Bioinformatics.

9.4 ANALYSIS OF INTERACTION RESULT OBTAINED FROM MOLECULAR DOCKING

The molecular docking or molecular interaction analysis is proceeded for calculating the binding energy of receptor and ligand. To compute the key features of binding performance between three dimensional structure of cytochrome P450 3A4 protein with cyclohexane, 1,2,4-triethenyl- resulting in the binding energy -7.9 kcal/mol, in which the residues ILE50, TYR53, ARG106, PHE215, LEU216, PHE220, and LEU221 exhibit hydrophobic interactions. Ribbon structure representation of 5VCC with cyclohexane, 1,2,4-triethenyl- is shown in Figure 9.1. The ball and stick representation of cyclohexane, 1,2,4-triethenyl- with 5VCC is shown in Figure 9.2.

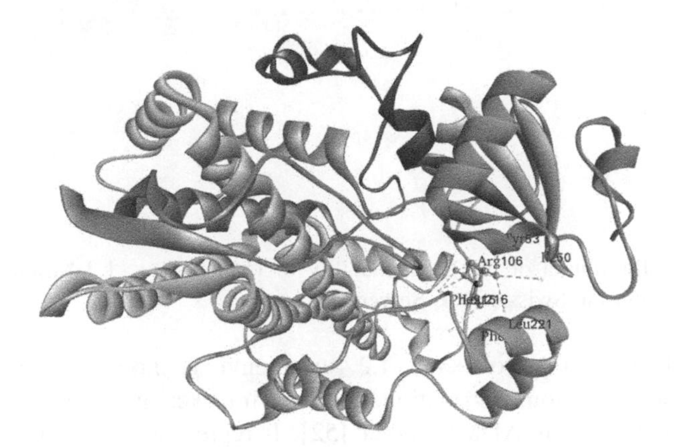

FIGURE 9.1 Ribbon Structure Representation of 5VCC with Cyclohexane, 1,2,4-triethenyl-. This Interaction Figure was Created with the Help of AutoDock Vina 4.2 [49], Pymol Visualizer Software [50], and Discovery Studio Visualize Software [51].

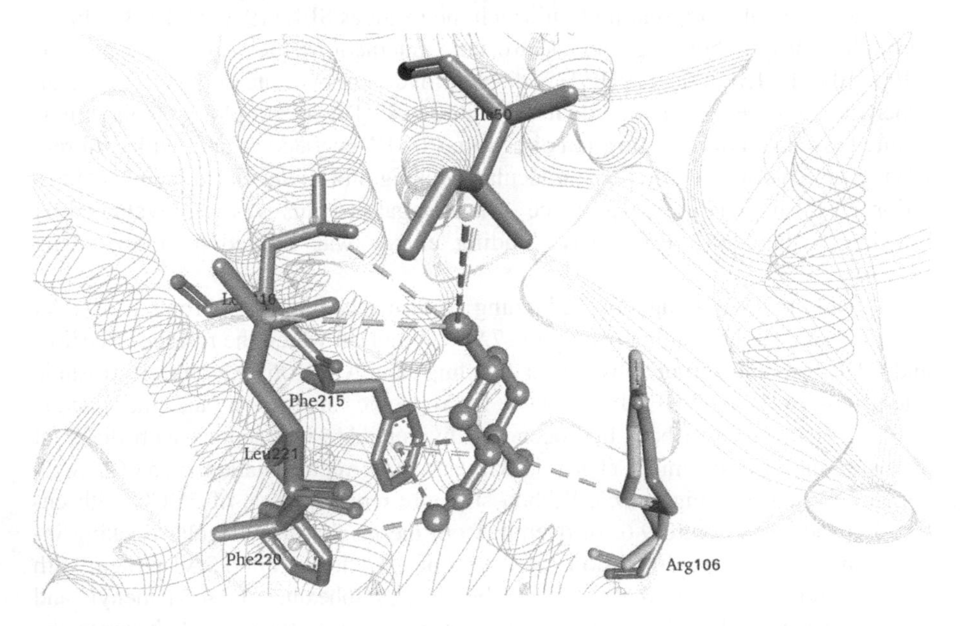

FIGURE 9.2 Ball and Stick Representation of Cyclohexane, 1,2,4-triethenyl- with 5VCC. This Interaction Figure was Created with the Help of AutoDock Vina 4.2 [49], Pymol Visualizer Software [50], and Discovery Studio Visualize Software [51].

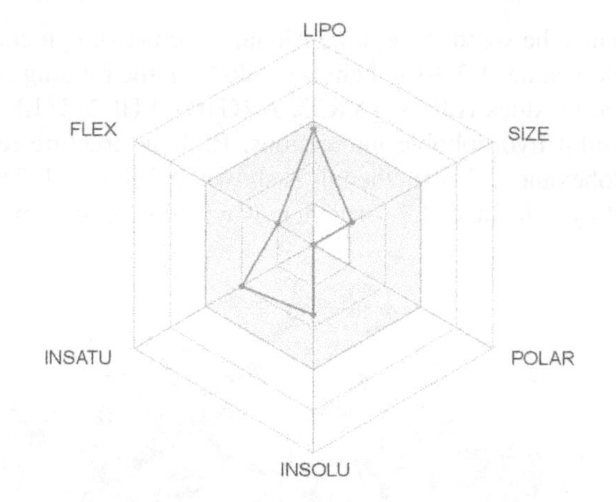

FIGURE 9.3 Illustration of the Bioavailability of Cyclohexane, 1,2,4-triethenyl-. Figure was Obtained by using SwissADME Server [52].

The bioavailability of cyclohexane, 1,2,4-triethenyl- is shown in Figure 9.3. It is noted that, the absorption, distribution, metabolisim, excreation (ADME) properties were evaluated by SwissADME server [52]. It represents the properties of lipophilicity, size, polarity, water solubility, insaturation, and flexibility. The pink color area is within the range of all properties. The radar plot of cyclohexane, 1,2,4-triethenyl- satisfies the properties of drug likeness.

The binding performance between studied protein with apigenin results in the binding energy of -10.5 kcal/mol, in which the residues SER119 and GLU374 binds through hydrogen bonding and electrostatic interactions, respectively, where as ARG 105, PHE108, and PHE215 display hydrophobic interaction. The detail schematic representation is shown in Figure 9.4. The radar plot of apigenin is pointed towards more in saturation direction. PLCE1-encoded protein with different phytochemicals was studied by molecular docking and molecular dynamics simulation [53]. The binding performance of antifungal proteins was also evaluated by docking method [54]. Previously, binding energy was studied by the docking process [55–57].

Similarly in case of eugenol the binding performance with cytochrome p450 3A4 protein results in the binding energy of -7.9 kcal/mol. In which the residues PHE215 and THR224 bind through hydrogen bonding and ARG106 exhibits electrostatic interaction, whereas PHE108 displays hydrophobic interaction and the residue PHE215 is involved in both hydrogen and hydrophobic interactions with different atoms of the phytochemical eugenol. Ball and stick representation of 5VCC with eugenol is shown in Figure 9.5. Ribbon structure representation of 5VCC with eugenol is shown in Figure 9.6. In overall, from the results of molecular docking interaction between three-dimensional structure of cytochrome P450 3A4 protein with different molecules show that the phytochemical cyclohexane, 1,2,4-triethenyl- and apigenin have the best binding performance as compare to eugenol, because the binding affinity is high in case of cyclohexane, 1,2,4-triethenyl-and apigenin. Apigenin shows better drug-like binding with the studied protein compared to others.

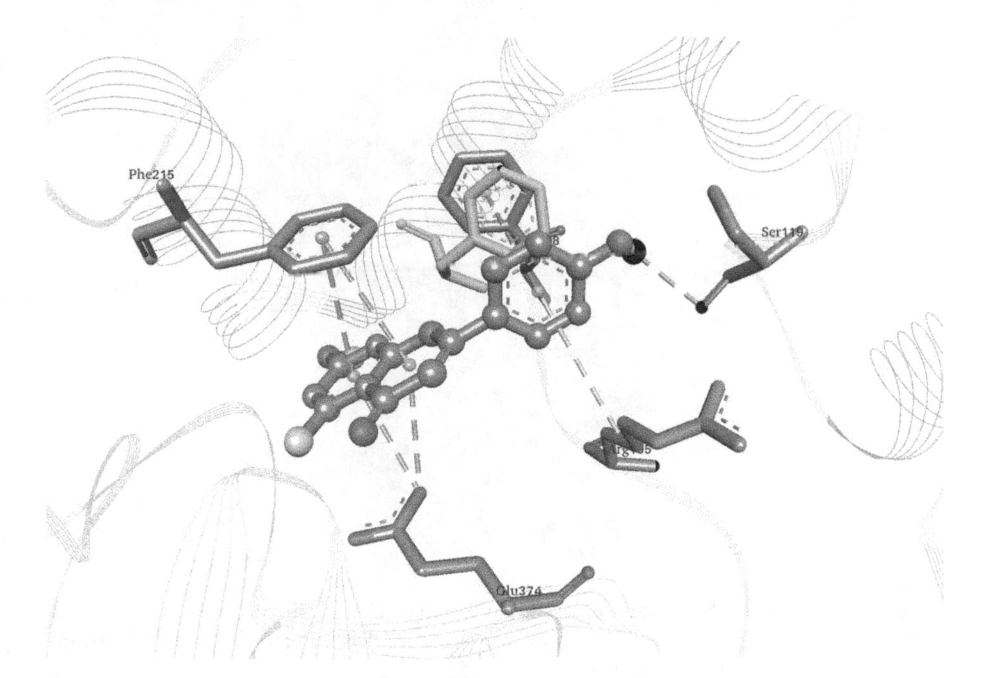

FIGURE 9.4 Ball and Stick Representation of Apigenin with 5VCC. This Interaction Figure was Created with the Help of AutoDock Vina 4.2 [49], Pymol Visualizer Software [50], and Discovery Studio Visualize Software [51].

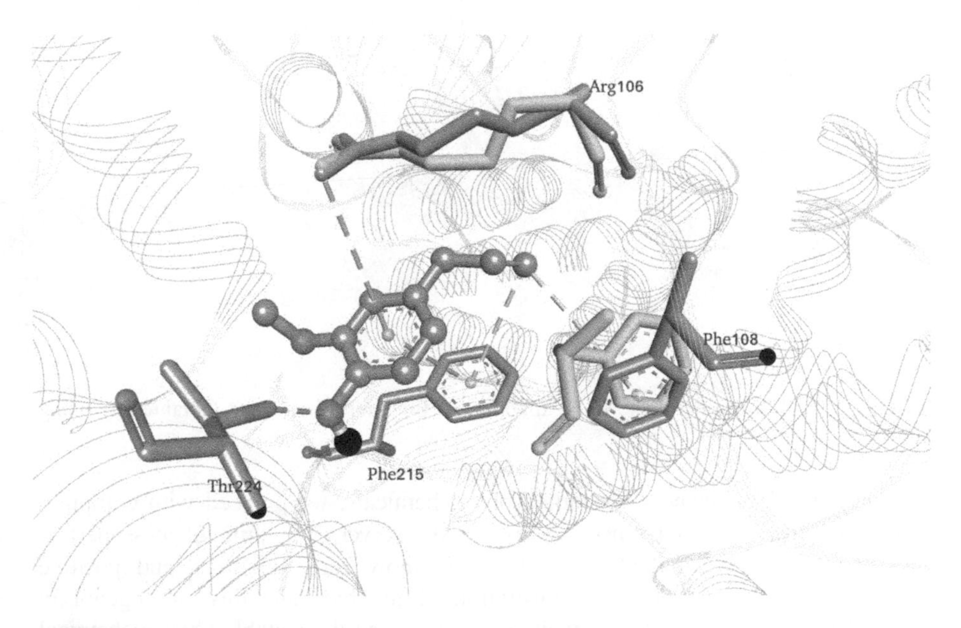

FIGURE 9.5 Ball and Stick Representation of 5VCC with Eugenol. This Interaction Figure was Created with the Help of AutoDock Vina 4.2 [49], Pymol Visualizer Software [50], and Discovery Studio Visualize Software [51].

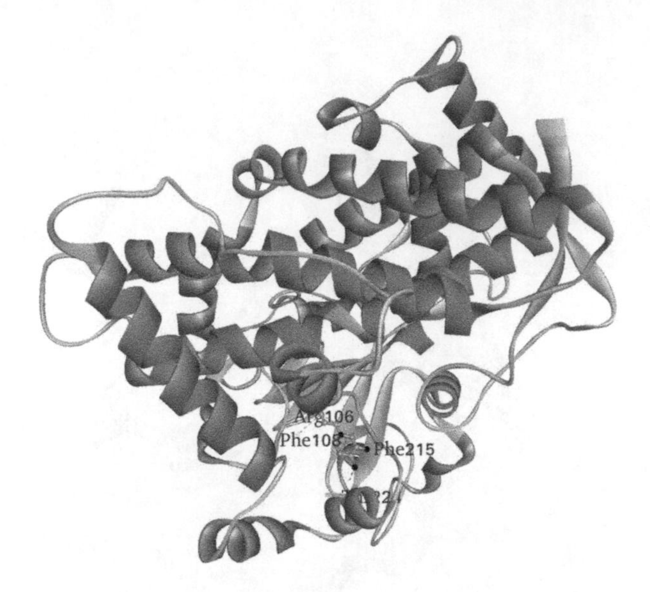

FIGURE 9.6 Ribbon Structure Representation of 5VCC with Eugenol. This Interaction Figure was Created with the Help of AutoDock Vina 4.2 [49], Pymol Visualizer Software [50], and Discovery Studio Visualize Software [51].

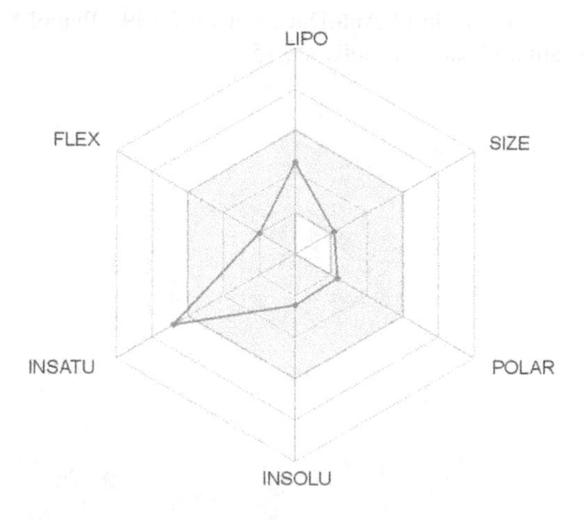

FIGURE 9.7 Illustration of the Bioavailability of Eugenol. Figure was Obtained by using SwissADME Server [34].

To verify the drug likeness of studied phytochemicals, we proceed with computational drug likeness test by using SwissADME server. The drug likeness performances of the three studied phytochemicals show zero violations and positive response towards drug likeness. Illustration of the bioavailability of eugenol in Figure 9.7. The red-colored part of the graph showing the suitable physicochemical space for oral bioavailability and our studied compounds also fall in the colored region. The binding energy is higher as compared to both the other studied molecules.

TABLE 9.1
Name of Phytochemicals, Binding Energies, Residues Involve During Interactions and Properties of Drug Likeness

Phytochemical name	Pubchem Id	Binding energy (kcal/ mol)	Binding residues	Types of bond/ interaction	Drug likeness
Cyclohexane, 1,2,4-triethenyl-	96529	−7.9	UNK0:C - A:PHE215	Hydrophobic	Yes:0
			violation		
			UNK0:C - A:ARG106	Hydrophobic	
			UNK0:C - A:ILE50	Hydrophobic	
			UNK0:C - A:LEU216	Hydrophobic	
			UNK0:C - A:LEU221	Hydrophobic	
			TYR53 -:UNK0:C	Hydrophobic	
			PHE215 -:UNK0:C	Hydrophobic	
			PHE215 -:UNK0:C	Hydrophobic	
PHE220 -:UNK0:C	Hydrophobic				
Apigenin	5280443	−10.5	UNK0:H - A:SER119:O	Hydrogen Bond	Yes:0
			violation		
			GLU374:OE1 -:UNK0	Electrostatic	
			GLU374:OE1 -:UNK0	Electrostatic	
			PHE108 -:UNK0	Hydrophobic	
			PHE215 -:UNK0	Hydrophobic	
			PHE215 -:UNK0	Hydrophobic	
UNK0 - A:ARG105	Hydrophobic				
Eugenol	3314	−7.3	THR224:OG1-:UNK0:O	Hydrogen Bond	Yes:0
			violation		
			UNK0:H - A:PHE215:O	Hydrogen Bond	
			ARG106:NH1 -:UNK0	Electrostatic	
			PHE215 -:UNK0	Hydrophobic	
			PHE108 -:UNK0:C	Hydrophobic	
PHE215 -:UNK0:C	Hydrophobic				

From the overall results of molecular docking and drug likeness test, the apigenin and eugenol show the best inhibitory effect as compared to cyclohexane, 1,2,4-triethenyl- because of hydrogen bonding and electrostatic interaction as well as negative binding affinity. The detailed results are shown in Table 9.1.

9.5 SUMMARY AND CONCLUSIONS

By addressing problems such as aging population-related diseases and autoimmune disorders, rising chronic disease incidence day-by-day, and people's expectations for more affordable and effective solutions, bioinformatics approaches will significantly benefit healthcare providers. Bioinformatics is now a relevant subject because of its healthcare potential, which relies on the ability to evaluate decision-making trends and derive knowledge of prescription drugs. People do not meet the needs of their complex diseases because of the limited resources of healthcare system in rural areas. In this modern period, the contribution of IoT to big data analysis is very important and appreciable [58]. Big data scanning helps extract vital data for applications in various fields, such as agriculture, manufacturing, and healthcare system. In the healthcare sector, the opportunities of big data research are to handle the vast volume of data being used to optimize patient care and to add value to healthcare services [59]. These diseases are essentially related to long-term illnesses and become serious over time. Other variables such as stress, diet, infection also lead to this condition. In traditional medicine, different parts of tulsi plant have been recommended for the treatment of bronchitis, diabetes, arthritis, cancer, autoimmune disorders, and various aging-related diseases. In this chapter, we have carried out molecular docking study to evaluate the interactions of the phytochemicals like cyclohexane, 1,2,4-triethenyl-, apigenin, and eugenol from tulsi leaves with human cytochromes P450 3A4. Cytochrome P450 3A4 protein is expressed in different organs according to age, and they also affect the metabolic function of other proteins. In cytochrome p450 3A4 protein with cyclohexane, 1,2,4-triethenyl- interaction, the residues ILE50, TYR53, ARG106, PHE215, LEU216, PHE220, and LEU221 exhibit hydrophobic interaction. Protein with apigenin interaction, the residues SER119 and GLU374 bind through hydrogen bonding and electrostatic interactions, respectively, whereas ARG105, PHE108, and PHE215 display hydrophobic interaction. The binding energies of phytochemicals with protein were predicted by using molecular docking study and found that the binding energies were -7.9, -10.5, and -7.3 kcal/mol for cyclohexane, 1,2,4-triethenyl-, apigenin, and eugenol, respectively. These computational outcomes are considered significant and innovative such that they can overcome the shortcomings of traditional healthcare system with the help of different bioinformatics and computational approaches.

REFERENCES

[1]. D. Lupton, Critical perspectives on digital health technologies. *Sociology Compass*, 8 (2014): 1344–1359.

[2]. U. Sivarajah, M.M. Kamal, Z. Irani, V. Weerakkody, Critical analysis of big data challenges and analytical methods. *Journal of Business Research*, 70 (2017): 263–286.

[3]. P.P. Reid, W.D. Compton, J.H. Grossman, G. Fanjiang, Information and communications systems: The backbone of the health care delivery system. In *Building a Better Delivery System: A New Engineering/Health Care Partnership*. National Academies Press, 2005.

[4]. M. Molaei, J. Sheng, Imaging bacterial 3D motion using digital in-line holographic microscopy and correlation-based de-noising algorithm. *Optics Express*, 22 (2014): 32119–32137.

[5]. R.B. Altman, R. Balling, J.F. Brinkley, E. Coiera, F. Consorti, M.A. Dhansay, A. Geissbuhler, W. Hersh, S.Y. Kwankam, N.M. Lorenzi, F. Martin-Sanchez, Commentaries on Informatics and medicine: From molecules to populations. *Methods of Information in Medicine*, 47 (2008): 296–317.

[6]. J. Guo, B. Li, The application of medical artificial intelligence technology in rural areas of developing countries. *Health Equity*, 2 (2018): 174–181.

[7]. A. Sharma, R.A. Harrington, M. B. McClellan, M.P. Turakhia, Z.J. Eapen, S. Steinhubl, J.R. Mault, M.D. Majmudar, L. Roessig, K. J. Chandross, E. M. Green, Using digital health technology to better generate evidence and deliver evidence-based care. *Journal of the American College of Cardiology*, 71 (2018): 2680–2690.

[8]. D.W. Bates, S. Saria, L. Ohno-Machado, A. Shah, G. Escobar, Big data in health care: Using analytics to identify and manage high-risk and high-cost patients. *Health Affairs*, 33(2014): 1123–1131.

[9]. D.B. Pisoni, W.G. Kronenberger, M.S. Harris, A.C. Moberly, Three challenges for future research on cochlear implants. *World Journal of Otorhinolaryngology - Head and Neck Surgery*, 3 (2017): 240–254.

[10]. M.R. Schmeler, R.M. Schein, M. McCue, K. Betz, Telerehabilitation clinical and vocational applications for assistive technology: Research, opportunities, and challenges. *International Journal of Telerehabilitation*, 1 (2009): 59.

[11]. M.E. Johnston, K.B. Langton, R.B. Haynes, A. Mathieu, Effects of computer-based clinical decision support systems on clinician performance and patient outcome: A critical appraisal of research. *Annals of Internal Medicine*, 120 (1994): 135–142.

[12]. G. Rong, A. Mendez, E.B. Assi, B. Zhao, M. Sawan, Artificial intelligence in healthcare: Review and prediction case studies. *Engineering*, 6 (2020): 291–301.

[13]. B. Davie, V. Florance, A. Friede, J. Sheehan, J.E. Sisk, Bringing health-care applications to the internet. *IEEE Internet Computing*, 5 (2001): 42–48.

[14]. C.L. Ventola, Mobile devices and apps for health care professionals: Uses and benefits. *Journal of Clinical Pharmacy and Therapeutics*, 39 (2014): 356.

[15]. W. Raghupathi, V. Raghupathi, Big data analytics in healthcare: Promise and potential. *Health Information Science and Systems*, 2 (2014): 3.

[16]. S. Jabbar, F. Ullah, S. Khalid, M. Khan, K. Han, Semantic interoperability in heterogeneous IoT infrastructure for healthcare. *Wireless Communications and Mobile Computing*, 2017 (2017): 9731806.

[17]. I. Chiuchisan, H.N. Costin, O. Geman, Adopting the internet of things technologies in health care systems. In *2014 International Conference and Exposition on Electrical and Power Engineering (EPE)* (pp. 532–535). IEEE, 2014.

[18]. S.R. Islam, D. Kwak, M.H. Kabir, M. Hossain, K.S. Kwak, The internet of things for health care: A comprehensive survey. *IEEE Access*, 3 (2015): 678–708.

[19]. U. Padhye, Excess dietary iron is the root cause for increase in childhood autism and allergies. *Medical Hypotheses*, 61 (2003): 220–222.

[20]. A. Sudhakar, History of cancer, ancient and modern treatment methods. *Journal of Cancer Science & Therapy*, 1 (2009): 1–4.

[21]. C. Robert, T. S. Kupper, Inflammatory skin diseases, T cells, and immune surveillance. *New England Journal of Medicine*, 341 (1999): 1817–1828.

[22]. A. Siebecker, Traditional bone broth in modern health and disease. *Townsend Letter for Doctors and Patients*, (2005): 74–82.

[23]. D.A. Smith, D.R. Germolec, Introduction to immunology and autoimmunity. *Environmental Health Perspectives*, 107 (1999): 661–665.

[24]. D.E. Trentham, R.A. Dynesius-Trentham, E.J. Orav, D. Combitchi, C. Lorenzo, K.L. Sewell, D.A. Hafler, H.L. Weiner, Effects of oral administration of type II collagen on rheumatoid arthritis. *Science*, 261 (1993): 1727–1730.

[25]. J.S. Smolen, K. Redlich, J. Zwerina, D. Aletaha, G. Steiner, G. Schett, Pro-inflammatory cytokines in rheumatoid arthritis. *Clinical Reviews in Allergy & Immunology*, 28 (2005): 239–248.

[26]. A. Fasano, Surprises from celiac disease. *Scientific American*, 301 (2009): 54–61.

[27]. C. Catassi, A. Fasano, Celiac disease. In *Gluten-Free Cereal Products and Beverages* (pp. 1–I). Academic Press, 2008.

[28]. M.A. Atkinson, G.S. Eisenbarth, Type 1 diabetes: New perspectives on disease pathogenesis and treatment. *The Lancet*, 358 (2001): 221–229.

[29]. R.P. Robertson, Prevention of recurrent hypoglycemia in type 1 diabetes by pancreas transplantation. *Acta Diabetologica*, 36 (1999): 3–9.

[30]. K.D. Burman, L. McKinley-Grant, Dermatologic aspects of thyroid disease. *Clinics in Dermatology*, 24 (2006): 247–255.

[31]. R.C. Sergott, J.S. Glaser, Graves' ophthalmopathy. A clinical and immunologic review. *Survey of Ophthalmology*, 26 (1981): 1–21.

[32]. T. Bodenheimer, E.H. Wagner, K. Grumbach, Improving primary care for patients with chronic illness: The chronic care model, Part 2. *Jama*, 288 (2002): 1909–1914.

[33]. G.E. Demas, The energetics of immunity: A neuroendocrine link between energy balance and immune function. *Hormones and Behavior*, 45 (2004): 173–180.

[34]. N. Baumgarth, J.W. Tung, L.A. Herzenberg, Inherent specificities in natural antibodies: A key to immune defense against pathogen invasion. In *Springer Seminars in Immunopathology* (vol. 26, no. 4, pp. 347–362). Springer-Verlag, 2005.

[35]. H. Pircher, U.H. Rohrer, D. Moskophidis, R.M. Zinkernagel, H. Hengartner, Lower receptor avidity required for thymic clonal deletion than for effector T-cell function. *Nature*, 351 (1991): 482.

[36]. S.B. Kirton, C.W. Murray, M.L. Verdonk, R.D. Taylor, Prediction of binding modes for ligands in the cytochromes P450 and other heme-containing proteins. *Proteins: Structure, Function, and Bioinformatics*, 58 (2005): 836–844.

[37]. T.A. Hennen-Bierwagen, Q. Lin, F. Grimaud, V. Planchot, P.L. Keeling, M.G. James, A.M. Myers, Proteins from multiple metabolic pathways associate with starch biosynthetic enzymes in high molecular weight complexes: A model for regulation of carbon allocation in maize amyloplasts. *Plant Physiology*, 149 (2009): 1541–1559.

[38]. J.L. Ferrer, M.B. Austin, C. Stewart Jr, J.P. Noel, Structure and function of enzymes involved in the biosynthesis of phenylpropanoids. *Plant Physiology and Biochemistry*, 46 (2008): 356–370.

[39]. D.V. Parke, *The Biochemistry of Foreign Compounds: International Series of Monographs in Pure and Applied Biology: Biochemistry* (vol. 5). Elsevier, 2013.

[40]. M. Ingelman-Sundberg, Polymorphism of cytochrome P450 and xenobiotic toxicity. *Toxicology*, 181 (2002): 447–452.

[41]. K. Lown, J. Kolars, K. Turgeon, R. Merion, S.A. Wrighton, P.B. Watkins, The erythromycin breath test selectively measures P450IIIA in patients with severe liver disease. *Clinical Pharmacology & Therapeutics*, 51 (1992): 229–238.

[42]. C.A. Gutekunst, A.I. Levey, C.J. Heilman, W.L. Whaley, H. Yi, N.R. Nash, H.D. Rees, J.J. Madden, S.M. Hersch, Identification and localization of huntingtin in brain and human lymphoblastoid cell lines with anti-fusion protein antibodies. *Proceedings of the National Academy of Sciences*, 92 (1995): 8710–8714.

[43]. C.M. Croce, P.C. Nowell, Molecular basis of human B cell neoplasia. In *RNA Tumor Viruses, Oncogenes, Human Cancer and AIDS: On the Frontiers of Understanding*(pp. 116–126). Springer, 1985.

[44]. D.M. Engman, J.S. Leon, Pathogenesis of Chagas heart disease: Role of autoimmunity. *Acta Tropica*, 81 (2002): 123–132.
[45]. Z. Wen, C. Fiocchi, Inflammatory bowel disease: Autoimmune or immune-mediated pathogenesis?. *Journal of Immunology Research*, 11 (2004): 195–204.
[46]. A. Chand, P. Chettiyankandy, M. Moharana, S.N. Sahu, S.K. Pradhan, S.K. Pattanayak, S.P. Mahapatra, A. Bissoyi, A.K. Singh, S. Chowdhuri, Computational methods for developing novel antiaging interventions. In *Molecular Basis and Emerging Strategies for Anti-aging Interventions* (pp. 175–193). Springer, 2018.
[47]. G. Devendran, U. Balasubramanian, Qualitative phytochemical screening and GC-MS analysis of Ocimum sanctum L. leaves. *Asian Journal of Plant Science and Research*, 1 (2011): 44–48.
[48]. M.S. Baliga, R. Jimmy, K.R. Thilakchand, V. Sunitha, N.R. Bhat, E. Saldanha, S. Rao, P. Rao, R. Arora, P.L. Palatty, Ocimum sanctum L (Holy Basil or Tulsi) and its phytochemicals in the prevention and treatment of cancer. *Nutrition and Cancer*, 65 (2013): 26–35.
[49]. X.Y. Meng, H.X. Zhang, M. Mezei, M. Cui, Molecular docking: A powerful approach for structure-based drug discovery. *Current Computer-Aided Drug Design*, 7 (2011): 146–157.
[50]. W.L. DeLano, Pymol: An open-source molecular graphics tool. *CCP4 Newsletter on Protein Crystallography*, 40 (2002): 82–92.
[51]. D.S. Visualizer, *Version 2.0. 1.7347.* Accelrys Software Inc., 2013.
[52]. A. Daina, O. Michielin, V. Zoete, SwissADME: A free web tool to evaluate pharmacokinetics, drug-likeness and medicinal chemistry friendliness of small molecules. *Scientific Reports*, 7 (2017): 42717.
[53]. S.N. Sahu, S.K. Pattanayak, Molecular docking and molecular dynamics simulation studies on PLCE1 encoded protein. *Journal of Molecular Structure*, 1198 (2019): 126936.
[54]. S.N. Sahu, M. Moharana, R. Sahu, S.K. Pattanayak, Molecular docking approach study of binding performance of antifungal proteins. In *AIP Conference Proceedings* (vol. 2142, no. 1, pp. 060001). AIP Publishing, 2019.
[55]. S.N. Sahu, M. Moharana, S.R. Martha, A. Bissoyi, P.K. Maharana, S.K. Pattanayak, Computational biology approach in management of big data of healthcare sector. In *Big Data Analytics for Intelligent Healthcare Management* (pp. 247–267). Academic Press, 2019.
[56]. J. Panda, J.K. Sahoo, P.K. Panda, S.N. Sahu, M. Samal, S.K. Pattanayak, R. Sahu, Adsorptive behavior of zeolitic imidazolate framework-8 towards anionic dye in aqueous media: Combined experimental and molecular docking study. *Journal of Molecular Liquids*, 278 (2019): 536–545.
[57]. S.N. Sahu, M. Moharana, R. Sahu, S.K. Pattanayak, Impact of mutation on podocin protein involved in type 2 nephrotic syndrome: Insights into docking and molecular dynamics simulation study. *Journal of Molecular Liquids*, 281 (2019): 549–562.
[58]. M.G. Sarowar, M.S. Kamal, N. Dey, Internet of things and its impacts in computing intelligence: A comprehensive review–IoT application for big data. In *Big Data Analytics for Smart and Connected Cities* (pp. 103–136). IGI Global, 2019.
[59]. N. Dey, A.E. Hassanien, C. Bhatt, A. Ashour, S.C. Satapathy, eds., *Internet of Things and Big Data Analytics Toward Next-Generation Intelligence* (pp. 3–549). Springer, 2018.

10 Aspects of Improvement of Digital Healthcare Systems Through Digital Transformation

Maheswata Moharana[1], Satya Narayan Sahu[2], Subrat Kumar Pattanayak[1], and Fahmida Khan[1]
[1]Department of Chemistry, National Institute of Technology, Raipur, India
[2]School of Applied Sciences, Kalinga Institute of Industrial Technology, Deemed to be University, Bhubaneswar, India

CONTENTS

10.1 INTRODUCTION: DIGITAL TRANSFORMATION IN HEALTHCARE SYSTEM

Digital health technology offers an interesting opportunity to improve clinical research along with the delivery of clinical care by enhancing quality, effectiveness, accessibility, protection, and personalization [1]. The digital health system, which is broadly defined, uses information, data, and communication technologies to collect, communicate, and analyze health information to enhance patient health [2]. The digital health system is also limited to electronic health, i.e., health records, facilities, and services that can be supplied electronically [3]. The future applications of digital health technology are to accelerate and simplify clinical research operations, while minimizing costs and allowing innovations to make traditional randomized clinical trials simpler and more advanced [4]. Healthcare organizations in both the private and public sectors are now moving very quickly towards full digitalization in a rapidly growing society. Healthcare organization strengthens their structures by digitalizing their products, services, and processes for the sake of change [5]. Digital health innovations may contribute to improving access to health services, lowering

DOI: 10.1201/9781003198796-10

costs, improving the quality of care, improving the efficacy of health systems, and even creating self-care opportunities. Remote tracking systems and wearable devices, for instance, help people maintain better health [6]. This technology is being used in telemedicine, various wearable devices, artificial intelligence, and genomics. Genomics is the field of molecular biology focused on an individual's genome sequencing data for diagnosis of diseases [7–9]. The term digital health should not be described as a clear-cut treatment tool, but it could be a way of bridging the gaps in the current healthcare system. It also offers the advantage of increasing access to underserved communities living in rural areas. From the point of view of protection, i.e., whether or not the digital health system is secure is a major concern for the common people. The best example mentioned in the previous study related to critical care medicine [10,11] can be used to explain this safety issue. While there is a beneficial association that links patient safety via digitalization devices, other technology should be enhanced at the same time, i.e., the quality of software program and algorithm creation in various apps. Healthcare services in every corner of the globe face a common problem, i.e., the need to develop affordable healthcare system. For example, drivers include rising demand among elderly people for chronic disease management, technical innovations, and allowing patients to have control over their health experience. In order to overcome these challenges, digital transformation in healthcare by technological advancements such as the Internet of Things, advanced analytics, machine learning, and artificial intelligence are well-known core components [12]. For the sake of system integration of patient data systems as well as cyber protection initiatives for networked medical equipment, the term digital transformation has emerged in the healthcare industry. This is the beneficial result of creativity in the healthcare system. Some of the significant examples of digital transformation in healthcare are telemedicine, artificial intelligence focused on medical instruments, and blockchain electronic health records. The proliferation of digital technologies will increase manufacturer trends in telemedicine, wearable devices, biometric sensors, clinical performance, and escalation of interoperability. From recent data, it was revealed that "Internet of Medical Things" will expand with spendings across all industries through digital transformation [13]. The extent of data generated by many sectors such as industrial, public administration, monetary sectors, and medical and scientific research has also increased infinitely due to increasing globalization. It can be revealed from many studies that 90% of the world's data produced is unstructured [14]. There is undeniably an era of big data in the picture to streamline these vast quantities of diverse and heterogeneous data. Big data is a technological phenomenon which through various formats such as social media, online transactions, e-commerce trends for future use, collects business information [15]. For the healthcare sector, it plays a key role. Healthcare markets, starting from single- and multi-provider organizations to large hospitals, are able to perceive substantial benefits by digitizing, merging, and using big data effectively. The benefits include early stage identification of diseases, minimization of prescription errors by patient record review, and promoting preventive treatment. Healthcare big data comes from both internal and external sources and also in different formats [16]. As healthcare costs are rising worldwide, certain common issues in traditional healthcare systems that are communicated face-to-face between the patient and the doctor continue to impact the experience of the patient. These concerns include access of physicians, prolonged waiting period, and unpleasantness of visits to the clinic and hospital [17]. In some developed countries, the waiting period to see a doctor can range from days to a month or even longer, where as in some countries many healthcare facilities are overcrowded with poor environments. It is often very difficult to have easy access to healthcare services through traditional healthcare delivery systems, especially in rural areas. In addition to this, visiting healthcare facilities is a costly affair in itself. In spite of the above issues, on-demand service networks, as in the transportation and hospitality sectors, have arisen in the healthcare industries. These networks concentrate predominantly on the services of primary care and consultation [18]. When considering this kind of content marketing, mobiles are particularly relevant. The on-demand healthcare platform enables patients to seek treatment from distributed physicians online. On these websites, doctors have registered either to be affiliated with local clinics and hospitals in order to provide such online services during their free time, or to perform services directly on the platforms. Physicians may also perform medical diagnoses, administer medications, and offer guidance and referrals to local health facilities. Virtual reality is based on computing technology that produces simulated or artificially three-dimensional environments that emulates reality [19]. It represents a strong interface that allows the user to realistically keep up with the computer-generated environment [20]. There are three types of virtual reality device (VR): interactive, semi-immersive, and non-immersive. Immersive systems are commonly known VR systems of the first form, where the consumer wears a head-mounted display . In the case of non-immersive VR, the user places a traditional graphics workstation in a three-dimensional environment that can be directly manipulated [21]. A virtual reality device offers very productive exposure to therapy when treating psychiatric patients suffering from specific anxiety disorder. A video screen that is positioned in front of the patient to view a picture of a particular graphical environment is characterized by this type of device. The display of the graphical environment on the video screen, the monitoring of the headset sensor to determine the location of the patient's head, and the manipulation of the graphical environment displayed on the video screen to represent the motion and position of the patient's head can also be managed by a computer programme that controls the operation of the device [22].

10.2 CHALLENGES OF DIGITAL TRANSFORMATION IN HEALTHCARE

Digital transformation is about transforming the way companies think and operate, by definition. There is a need for a change in attitude, beyond investing in modern technologies. Everybody needs to be on the same page, right from the doctors to the nurses and other hospital staff. In an effective digital transformation journey, coping with the all-too-familiar fear of change is the first and most critical challenge [23]. Healthcare companies prefer to concentrate on return on investment without fully realizing the value proposition that can be provided by a digitally driven infrastructure. It is wise to take into consideration the money saved, instead of looking at the expense incurred, until inefficient processes are remedied through digital transformation. Telemedicine will eliminate the need for in-person appointments, allowing more patients to be catered to by physicians. Similarly, going digital can be a real money-saver when it comes to chronic disease management [24]. The threat of cyberattacks comes with technology. For all technology-driven sectors, it is a massive challenge, but more so for healthcare, considering the sensitive and personal nature of the data involved [25]. Many healthcare firms are so afraid of the consequences that they refuse to take the digital plunge. Experts agree that in a digital world, there are myriad ways for organizations to ensure that patient data and study data are secure. Cyber security needs to become a top agenda, for instance. Companies need to invest in workers with the right skill set, inform staff on safety precautions, upgrade identified weaknesses in software, and ensure that systems and processes are built safely. Security measures need to be continuously updated in the ever-changing digital world to keep cyber threats in place [26]. Data is knowledge and power is knowledge. The amount of data produced on a day-to-day basis by healthcare organizations is immense, but very few can use it intelligently. For healthcare providers, data aggregation and interoperability are major challenges [27]. It is hard to collect, grasp, and act on available insights when data is trapped in silos around the organization. The dilemma cannot be solved by simply incorporating a fresh technology that many organizations mistake digital transformation to be [28]. Healthcare organizations must concentrate on incorporating data from all processes and promote cross-functional cooperation in order to make a holistic patient-centered perspective a reality. The challenge needs to be tackled from the top down; this battle cannot be fought by the IT department alone [29]. Thanks to the adoption of the integrated Hospital Information System (HIS) and electronic medical records, many hospitals claim to be "digital" today (EMR) [30]. Organizations need to understand a clear vision of how they will meet the digital needs of their clients, set goals against that vision, and then start executing it. The master plan must cover everything from investing in the necessary digital talent and modernizing existing systems, to offering real-time solutions and addressing security issues [31].

10.3 COMPUTER-AIDED DRUG DESIGN WITH H2N2 INFLUENZA A VIRUS

Influenza is a respiratory illness caused by the influenza virus. All of these symptoms typically begin and continue for up to a week. The most important human respiratory pathogens that cause both seasonal and endemic infections are these viruses. There have been a dozen of influenza A virus pandemics [32,33]. Because of its rapid transmission and high mortality rate, influenza is considered to be a prominent health concern. The family of orthomyxoviridae is associated with these influenza viruses [34]. Influenza A viruses are ecologically active pathogens that infect the host species extensively and that cause pandemics periodically in the human body [35]. Using nucleic acid protein inhibitors, neuraminidase inhibitors, and ion channel blockers, the disease was initially cured [36]. For antiviral therapies, the neuraminidase enzyme provides a seductive target. As stated in several literatures [37], this neuraminidase inhibition is an important and new idea in the treatment of influenza. Drugs are chemical substances that avoid illness or help recover the health of people who are sick. A chemical substance used in the treatment or prevention of illness or used to promote physical or mental well-being is a medicine in the pharmacological field. The presence of a certain concentration in the fluid binding to the target side of the host is necessary on the basis of the pharmacokinetic property of drug action. In other words, we can assume that the degree of the reaction depends on the drug concentration at the site of action. Any minimum pharmacokinetic properties, such as absorption, delivery, metabolism, excretion (ADME), and Lipinski, known as drug likeness, should be accompanied by a drug compound. By applying all these ideas, we can use computer techniques to design a drug compound. The computer-aided drug design for a drug molecule [38] is a time-consuming prediction. Some steps such as target identification, lead identification, binding side prediction, and prediction of ADME as well as drug similarity properties are followed by this technique. An example of computer-aided drug design for H2N2 influenza virus by targeting H2N2 virus neuraminidase protein by using computational methods and techniques is demonstrated in this current research. The three-dimensional neuraminidase structure was downloaded from a PDB database with PDB ID 1IVD from the protein data bank (PDB). The neuraminidase crystal structure resolution is 1.90 Å. The three-dimensional structure of the studied protein structure was analyzed using AutoDock Vina tools [39] to analyze the drug binding side with different phytocompounds and binding protein confirmations, and the process is called molecular interaction or molecular docking. It may be a protein-drug or two chemical compounds that are small molecules. The schematic representation is shown in Figure 10.1. In the docking phase of two molecules, one is taken as a receptor and another is treated as a

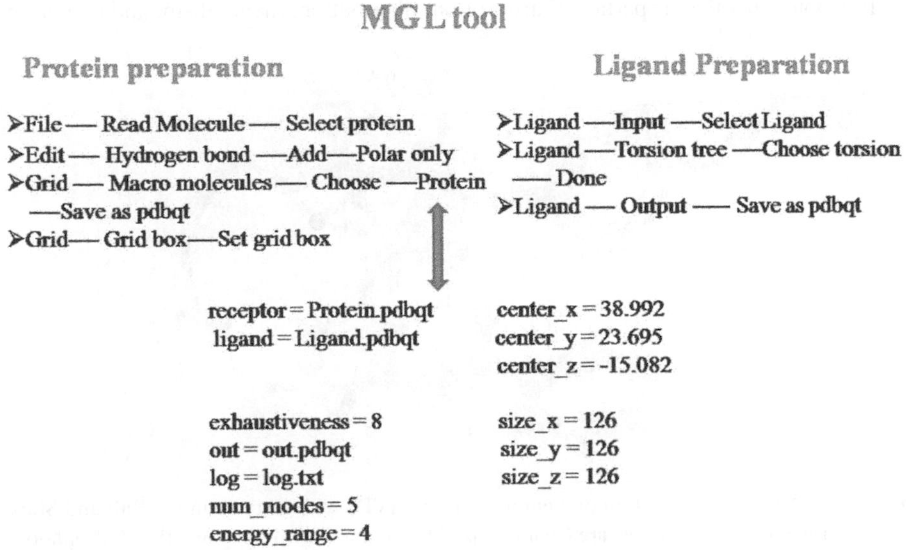

MGL tool

Protein preparation

➤File — Read Molecule — Select protein
➤Edit — Hydrogen bond —Add—Polar only
➤Grid — Macro molecules — Choose —Protein —Save as pdbqt
➤Grid— Grid box—Set grid box

Ligand Preparation

➤Ligand —Input —Select Ligand
➤Ligand —Torsion tree —Choose torsion — Done
➤Ligand — Output — Save as pdbqt

receptor = Protein.pdbqt
ligand = Ligand.pdbqt

center_x = 38.992
center_y = 23.695
center_z = -15.082

exhaustiveness = 8
out = out.pdbqt
log = log.txt
num_modes = 5
energy_range = 4

size_x = 126
size_y = 126
size_z = 126

FIGURE 10.1 Docking Workflow for Protein, Ligand and Grid Box Preparation. The Values of Center and Size are Provided for the Current Studied Receptor Using AutoDock Vina Tools [39].

ligand, in which we have to build a grid box on the receptor. The three-dimensional neuraminidase (1IVD) protein structure was taken as a receptor in the present research, and various pytochemicals such as chrysin [40], acacetin [41], and rotenone [42] are known as ligands. Using AutoDockTool version 1.5.6 [39], we measured the Kollman charges after removal of all bad contacts from the receptor and ligand and attached the hydrogen atoms to the polar contacts of the receptor. The autodock tool utilizes the gradient optimization algorithm during docking to perform the docking process. We fixed the grid box size of 126 × 126 × 126 in the direction of x, y, and z and center-x, center-y, center-z are respectively 38.992, 23.695, and -15.082 for the current studied receptor. The planning and visualization of the structure is carried out using Pymol Visualize software [43] and Visualize Discovery Studio software [44]. Following the interaction analysis, the computational drug similarity test for the phytochemicals tested was carried out using the Swiss ADME server [45].

10.4 ANALYSIS OF MOLECULAR INTERACTION

The binding energy of neuraminidase (receptor) and studied phytocompounds (ligand) is measured using molecular docking or molecular interaction analysis. To examine the main binding performance characteristics between the three-dimensional neuraminidase protein structure with chrysin, resulting in binding energy of -7.4 kcal/mol. Residue ARG420 binds through hydrogen bonding, while in hydrophobic interaction TYR284 interacts and in hydrophobic interaction ARG283 interacts with chrysin as well as hydrogen bonding to various chrysin atoms. The representation of neuraminidase and chrysin in the ball and sick model was shown in Figure 10.2. The bioavailability of chrysin demonstrated positive drug-like actions with a violation of 0. It is noted that the properties of absorption, distribution, metabolism, and excretion

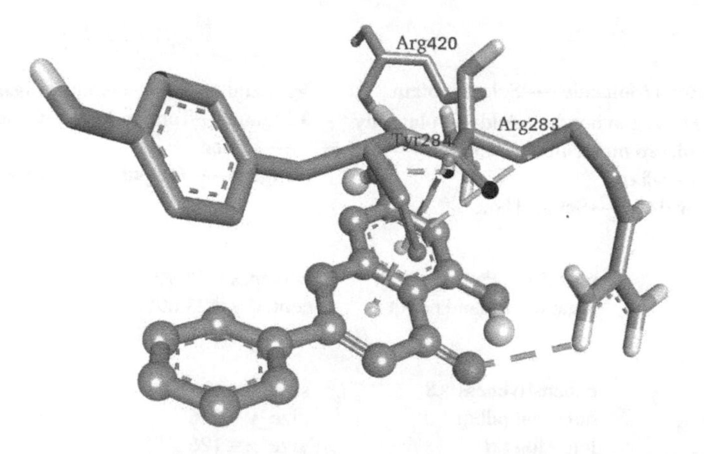

FIGURE 10.2 Representation of Neuraminidase (1IVD) with Chrysin in the Ball and Stick Model. The Gray Dotted Lines are Characterized by Hydrogen Bonding and the Hydrophobic Relationship is Represented by Pink Dotted Lines. Chrysin is the Ball and Stick Model and the Interacting Residues of 1IVD are Seen in Stick Models. With the Aid of AutoDock Vina [39], Pymol Visualizer Software [43], and Discovery Studio Visualization Software [44] this interaction figure was developed.

(ADME) were assessed using the SwissADME server [45]. The properties of lipophilicity, scale, polarity, solubility in water, instauration, and flexibility are described. The binding performance between studied protein with acacetin resulted in the binding energy of -6.7 kcal/mol, in which the residue THR148 binds through hydrogen bonding and ILE153, HIS150 interact in hydrophobic interactions. The detail schematic representation is shown in Figure 10.3. The phytocompound acacetin satisfies all the ADME properties for drug likeness, so it may be used as an inhibitor of neuraminidase, which is responsible for H2N2 influenza flu. Similarly, the binding efficiency of the binding energy is -7.1 kcal/mol in the case of rotenone with neuraminidase protein. In which the hydrogen bonding residues GLN91 and TRP383 are bonded. In both electrostatic and hydrophobic interactions, ASP355 and ILE418 residues interact. Ball and stick model representation of neuraminidase with rotenone is shown in Figure 10.4. The bioavailability of rotenone was showing positive respond towards drug likeness with 0 violation. Overall the results of the molecular docking interaction between three-dimensional neuraminidase protein structures with different molecules show that the phytocompound chrysin and rotenone have the best binding performance compared to acacetin, since in the case of chrysin and rotenone, the binding affinity is high. Compared to some, chrysin displays a stronger binding

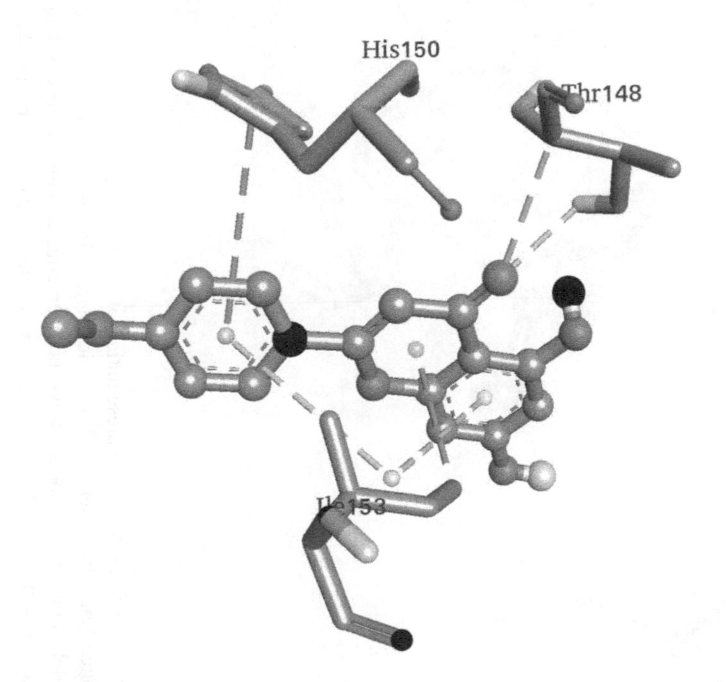

FIGURE 10.3 Ball and Stick Model Representation of Neuraminidase (1IVD) with Acacetin. The Dotted Gray Colored Lines Represent Hydrogen Bonding and Pink Dotted Lines Represent Hydrophobic Interaction. Acetin is the Ball and Stick Model and Stick Model Shows the Interacting Residues of 1IVD. This Interaction Figure was Created with the Help of AutoDock Vina [39], Pymol Visualizer Software [43], and Discovery Studio Visualize Software [44].

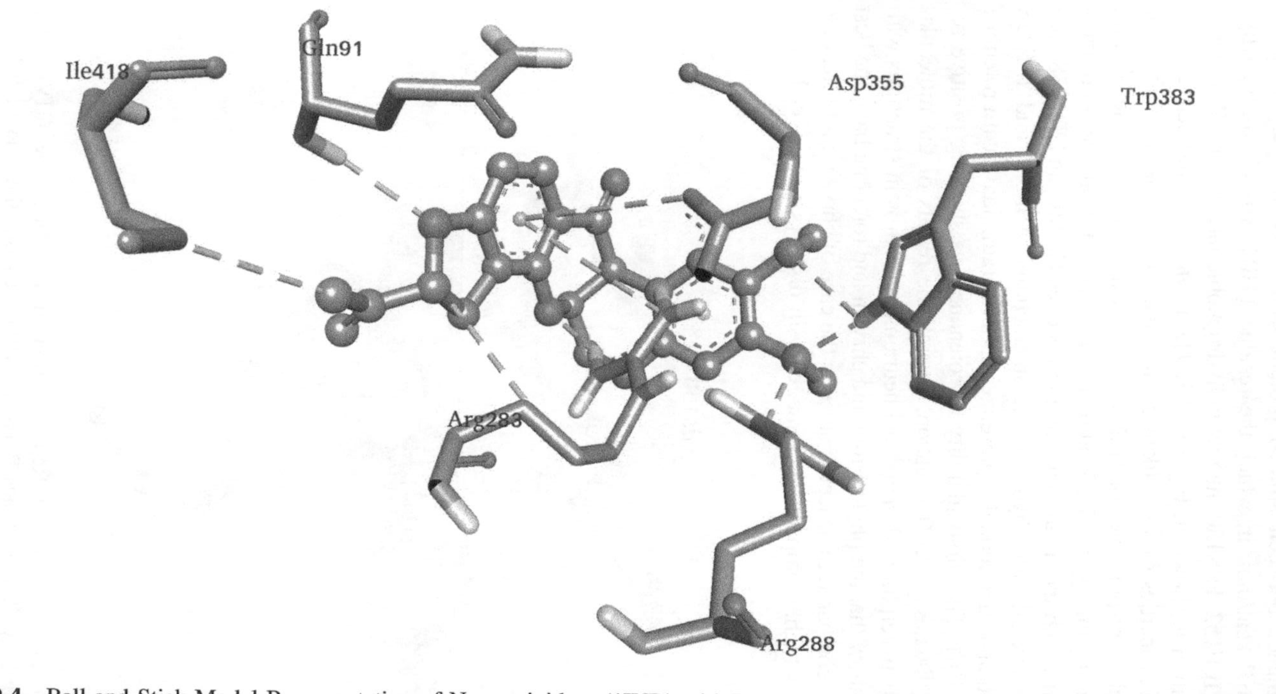

FIGURE 10.4 Ball and Stick Model Representation of Neuraminidase (1IVD) with Rotenone. The Dotted Gray Colored Lines Represent Hydrogen Bonding, Pink Dotted Lines Represent Hydrophobic Interaction, and the Yellow Dotted Lines Represent Electrostatic Interaction. Rotenone represents Ball and Stick Model and the Stick Model Shows the Interacting Residues of 1IVD. This Interaction Figure was Created with the Help of AutoDock Vina [39], Pymol Visualizer Software [43], and Discovery Studio Visualize Software [44].

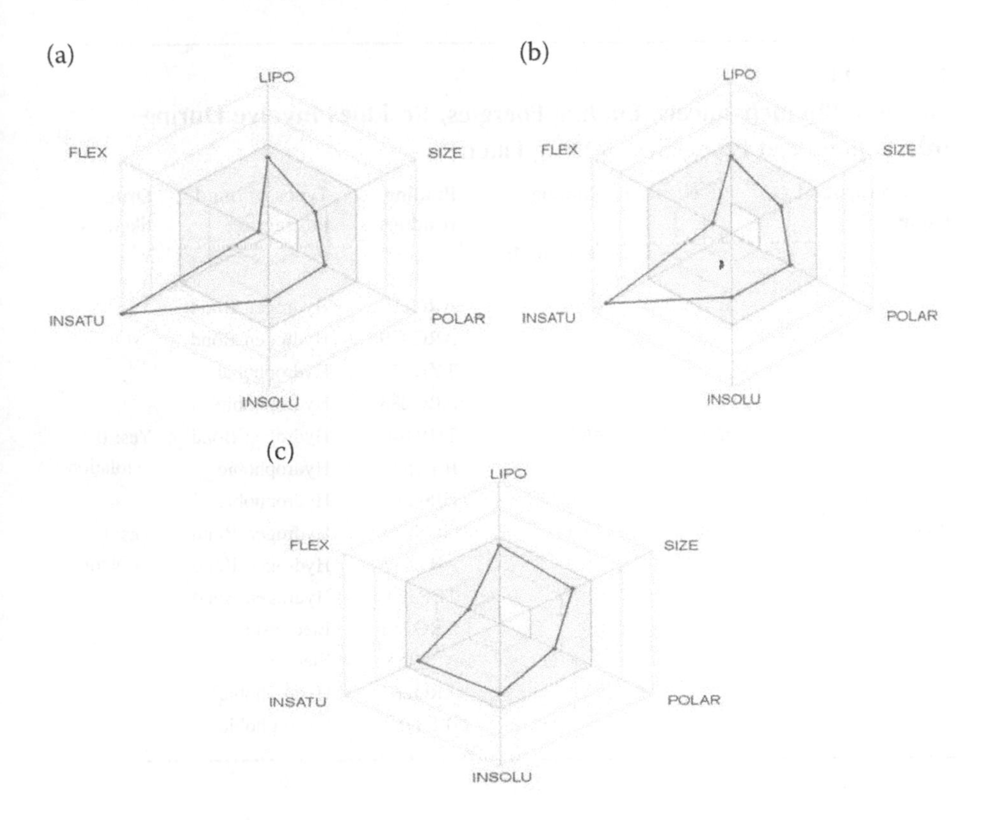

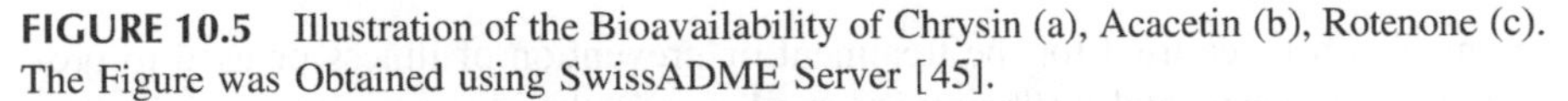

FIGURE 10.5 Illustration of the Bioavailability of Chrysin (a), Acacetin (b), Rotenone (c). The Figure was Obtained using SwissADME Server [45].

affinity, such as binding to the protein tested. The output of the three studied phytochemicals in drug likeness indicates zero violations and a positive response to drug likeness. Figure 10.5(a), (b), (c) is an example of the bioavailability and chemical structure of chrysin, acacetin, and rotenone. The physicochemical space for oral bioavailability is shown in the graph. The gray colored radar plot shows the oral bioavailability for our studied compounds in the side of the pink field. There are also decreases in the color area in our studied compounds. Overall, chrysin and rotenone display the best inhibitory activity compared to hydrogen bond acacetin and electrostatic interaction and negative binding affinity from the findings of the molecular docking and drug similarity analysis. The detailed result is shown in the Table 10.1.

10.5 SUMMARY AND CONCLUSIONS

Digital health innovations may contribute to improving access to health services, lowering costs, improving the quality of care, improving the efficacy of health systems, and even creating self-care opportunities. A key term used to explain the holistic impact generated by the implementation of digital technology is digital transformation and how that application radically transforms a specific domain. A

TABLE 10.1
Name of Phytochemicals, Binding Energies, Residues Involve During Interactions and Properties of Drug Likeness

Phytocompound name	Pubchem Id	Binding energy (kcal/mol)	Binding residues	Types of bond/ interaction	Drug likeness
Chrysin	5281607	−7.4	ARG283	Hydrogen Bond	Yes: 0 violation
			ARG420	Hydrogen Bond	
			TYR284	Hydrophobic	
			ARG283	Hydrophobic	
Acacetin	5280442	−6.7	THR148	Hydrogen Bond	Yes: 0 violation
			ILE153	Hydrophobic	
			HIS150	Hydrophobic	
Rotenone	6758	−7.1	GLN91	Hydrogen Bond	Yes: 0 violation
			ARG283	Hydrogen Bond	
			TRP383	Hydrogen Bond	
			ARG283	Electrostatic	
			ASP355	Electrostatic	
			ARG283	Hydrophobic	
			ILE418	Hydrophobic	

chemical substance used for the treatment or prevention of illness or used to promote physical or mental wellbeing is a medicine in the pharmacological field. The existence of a certain concentration in the fluid binding the target site of the host is dependent on the pharmacokinetic properties of drug action. Influenza viruses are ecologically active pathogens that infect a broad variety of host species and trigger pandemics that have periodically arisen in the human body. The virus can spread through the air from infected people's cough and sneeze. To examine the main binding performance characteristics between the three-dimensional neuraminidase protein structures with chrysin, resulting in the binding energy of -7.4 kcal/mol in which ARG420 residue binds through hydrogen bonding, while TYR284 interacts in hydrophobic interaction and ARG283 interacts in hydrophobic interaction with chrysin and hydrogen bonding. Similarly, the binding efficiency of the binding energy is -7.1 kcal/mol in the case of rotenone with neuraminidase protein. HIS150 engages in hydrophobic interactions. The binding output between the studied protein and acacetin was resulting in the binding energy of -6.7 kcal/mol, in which the residue THR148 bonds through hydrogen bonding and ILE153. Chrysin displays a stronger binding affinity. The output of the three studied phytochemicals in drug likeness indicates zero violations and a positive response to drug likeness.

REFERENCES

[1]. Murray, E., Hekler, E.B., Andersson, G., Collins, L.M., Doherty, A., Hollis, C., Rivera, D.E., West, R. and Wyatt, J.C., "Evaluating digital health interventions: key questions and approaches." American Journal of Preventive Medicine 51, no. 5 (2016): 843–851.

[2]. Sharma, A., Harrington, R.A., McClellan, M.B., Turakhia, M.P., Eapen, Z.J., Steinhubl, S., Mault, J.R., Majmudar, M.D., Roessig, L., Chandross, K.J. and Green, E.M., "Using digital health technology to better generate evidence and deliver evidence-based care." Journal of the American College of Cardiology 71, no. 23 (2018): 2680–2690.

[3]. Oh, H., Rizo, C., Enkin, M. and Jadad, A., "What is eHealth?: a systematic review of published definitions." World Hospitals and Health Services 41, no. 1 (2005): 32–40.

[4]. Fordyce, C.B., Roe, M.T., Ahmad, T., Libby, P., Borer, J.S., Hiatt, W.R., Bristow, M.R., Packer, M., Wasserman, S.M., Braunstein, N. and Pitt, B., "Cardiovascular drug development: is it dead or just hibernating?" Journal of the American College of Cardiology 65, no. 15 (2015): 1567–1582.

[5]. Khan, M.F.F. and Sakamura, K., "Fine-grained access control to medical records in digital healthcare enterprises." In 2015 International Symposium on Networks, Computers and Communications (ISNCC), pp. 1–6. IEEE, New Jersey, United States, 2015.

[6]. Gatzoulis, L. and Iakovidis, I., "Wearable and portable eHealth systems." IEEE Engineering in Medicine and Biology Magazine 26, no. 5 (2007): 51–56.

[7]. Panesar, A., "Future of healthcare." In Machine Learning and AI for Healthcare, pp. 255–304. Apress, Berkeley, CA, 2019.

[8]. Greaves, R.F., Bernardini, S., Ferrari, M., Fortina, P., Gouget, B., Gruson, D., Lang, T., Loh, T.P., Morris, H.A., Park, J.Y. and Roessler, M., "Key questions about the future of laboratory medicine in the next decade of the 21st century: a report from the IFCC-Emerging Technologies Division." Clinica Chimica Acta 495 (2019): 570–589.

[9]. Banerjee, A., Chakraborty, C., Kumar, A. and Biswas, D., "Emerging trends in IoT and big data analytics for biomedical and health care technologies." In Handbook of Data Science Approaches for Biomedical Engineering, pp. 121–152. Academic Press, Cambridge, 2020.

[10]. Agboola, S.O., Bates, D.W. and Kvedar, J.C., "Digital health and patient safety." Jama 315, no. 16 (2016): 1697–1698.

[11]. Lilly, C.M., Zubrow, M.T., Kempner, K.M., Reynolds, H.N., Subramanian, S., Eriksson, E.A., Jenkins, C.L., Rincon, T.A., Kohl, B.A., Groves Jr, R.H. and Cowboy, E.R., "Critical care telemedicine: evolution and state of the art." Critical Care Medicine 42, no. 11 (2014): 2429–2436.

[12]. Gopal, G., Suter-Crazzolara, C., Toldo, L. and Eberhardt, W., "Digital transformation in healthcare–architectures of present and future information technologies." Clinical Chemistry and Laboratory Medicine (CCLM) 57, no. 3 (2019): 328–335.

[13]. Faddis, A., "The digital transformation of healthcare technology management." Biomedical Instrumentation & Technology 52, no. s2 (2018): 34–38.

[14]. Gantz, J. and Reinsel, D., "The digital universe in 2020: big data, bigger digital shadows, and biggest growth in the far east." IDC iView: IDC Analyze the Future 2007(2012): 1–16.

[15]. Sivarajah, U., Kamal, M.M., Irani, Z. and Weerakkody, V., "Critical analysis of big data challenges and analytical methods." Journal of Business Research 70 (2017): 263–286.

[16]. Raghupathi, W. and Raghupathi, V., "Big data analytics in healthcare: promise and potential." Health Information Science and Systems 2, no. 1 (2014): 3.
[17]. Dedding, C., Van Doorn, R., Winkler, L. and Reis, R., "How will e-health affect patient participation in the clinic? A review of e-health studies and the current evidence for changes in the relationship between medical professionals and patients." Social Science & Medicine 72, no. 1 (2011): 49–53.
[18]. Liu, Y., Wang, X., Gilbert, S. and Lai, G., "Pricing, quality and competition at on-demand healthcare service platforms." SSRN 3253855 (2018).
[19]. Sisto, S.A., Forrest, G.F. and Glendinning, D., "Virtual reality applications for motor rehabilitation after stroke." Topics in Stroke Rehabilitation 8, no. 4 (2002): 11–23.
[20]. Schultheis, M.T. and Rizzo, A.A., "The application of virtual reality technology in rehabilitation." Rehabilitation Psychology 46, no. 3 (2001): 296.
[21]. Ma, M. and Zheng, H., "Virtual reality and serious games in healthcare." In Advanced Computational Intelligence Paradigms in Healthcare 6. Virtual Reality in Psychotherapy, Rehabilitation, and Assessment, pp. 169–192. Springer, Berlin, Heidelberg, 2011.
[22]. Hodges, L.F. and Rothbaum, B.O., "Virtual reality system for treating patients with anxiety disorders." U.S. Patent 6,012,926, issued January 11, 2000.
[23]. Fitzgerald, M., Kruschwitz, N., Bonnet, D. and Welch, M., "Embracing digital technology: a new strategic imperative." MIT Sloan Management Review 55, no. 2 (2014): 1.
[24]. Elton, J. and O'Riordan, A., Healthcare Disrupted: Next Generation Business Models and Strategies. John Wiley & Sons, United States, 2016.
[25]. Qadir, J., Ali, A., ur Rasool, R., Zwitter, A., Sathiaseelan, A. and Crowcroft, J., "Crisis analytics: big data-driven crisis response." Journal of International Humanitarian Action 1, no. 1 (2016): 1–21.
[26]. Stoneburner, G., Goguen, A. and Feringa, A., "Risk management guide for information technology systems." NIST Special Publication 800, no. 30 (2002): 800–830.
[27]. Wang, Y. and Hajli, N., "Exploring the path to big data analytics success in healthcare." Journal of Business Research 70 (2017): 287–299.
[28]. Arthur, L., Big Data Marketing: Engage Your Customers More Effectively and Drive Value. John Wiley & Sons, United States, 2013.
[29]. Weberg, D. and Davidson, S., "Patient-centered care, evidence, and innovation." Leadership for Evidence-Based Innovation in Nursing and Health Professions (2017): 111–142.
[30]. Hillestad, R., Bigelow, J., Bower, A., Girosi, F., Meili, R., Scoville, R. and Taylor, R., "Can electronic medical record systems transform health care? Potential health benefits, savings, and costs." Health Affairs 24, no. 5 (2005): 1103–1117.
[31]. Friess, P., Digitising the Industry-Internet of Things Connecting the Physical, Digital and Virtual Worlds. River Publishers, Denmark, 2016.
[32]. Morens, D.M. and Fauci, A.S., "The 1918 influenza pandemic: insights for the 21st century." The Journal of Infectious Diseases 195, no. 7 (2007): 1018–1028.
[33]. Taubenberger, J.K. and Morens, D.M., "The pathology of influenza virus infections." Annual Review of Pathology: Mechanisms of Disease 3 (2008): 499–522.
[34]. Kamal, R.P., Tosh, C., Pattnaik, B., Behera, P., Nagarajan, S., Gounalan, S., Shrivastava, N., Shankar, B.P. and Pradhan, H.K., "Analysis of the PB2 gene reveals that Indian H5N1 influenza virus belongs to a mixed-migratory bird sub-lineage possessing the amino acid lysine at position 627 of the PB2 protein." Archives of Virology 152, no. 9 (2007): 1637–1644.

[35]. Joseph, U., Linster, M., Suzuki, Y., Krauss, S., Halpin, R.A., Vijaykrishna, D., Fabrizio, T.P., Bestebroer, T.M., Maurer-Stroh, S., Webby, R.J. and Wentworth, D.E., "Adaptation of pandemic H2N2 influenza A viruses in humans." Journal of Virology 89, no. 4 (2015): 2442–2447.

[36]. Ahmad, A., Javed, M.R., Rao, A.Q. and Husnain, T., "Designing and screening of universal drug from neem (Azadirachta indica) and standard drug chemicals against influenza virus nucleoprotein." BMC Complementary and Alternative Medicine 16, no. 1 (2016): 519.

[37]. Oxford, J.S. and Lambkin, R., "Targeting influenza virus neuraminidase-a new strategy for antiviral therapy." Drug Discovery Today 3, no. 10 (1998): 448–456.

[38]. Gilson, M., "The physical basis of computer-aided drug design: assessing and advancing the accuracy of binding affinity calculations." In APS Meeting Abstracts. 2019.

[39]. Meng, X.Y., Zhang, H.X., Mezei, M. and Cui, M., "Molecular docking: a powerful approach for structure-based drug discovery." Current Computer-Aided Drug Design 7, no. 2 (2011): 146–157.

[40]. Mani, R. and Natesan, V., "Chrysin: sources, beneficial pharmacological activities, and molecular mechanism of action." Phytochemistry 145 (2018): 187–196.

[41]. Naithani, R., Mehta, R.G., Shukla, D., Chandersekera, S.N. and Moriarty, R.M., "Antiviral activity of phytochemicals: a current perspective." In Dietary Components and Immune Function, pp. 421–468. Humana Press, Totowa, NJ, 2010.

[42]. Takatsuki, A., Nakatani, N., Morimoto, M., Tamura, G., Matsui, M., Arima, K., Yamaguchi, I. and Misato, T., "Antiviral and antitumor antibiotics. XX. Effects of rotenone, deguelin, and related compounds on animal and plant viruses." Applied and Environmental Microbiology 18, no. 4 (1969): 660–667.

[43]. DeLano, W.L., "Pymol: an open-source molecular graphics tool." CCP4 Newsletter on Protein Crystallography 40, no. 1 (2002): 82–92.

[44]. Visualizer, D.S., Version 2.0. 1.7347. Accelrys Software Inc., San Diego, 2013.

[45]. Daina, A., Michielin, O. and Zoete, V., "SwissADME: a free web tool to evaluate pharmacokinetics, drug-likeness and medicinal chemistry friendliness of small molecules." Scientific Reports 7 (2017): 42717.

11 Automated Detection of COVID-19 Lesion in Lung CT Slices with VGG-UNet and Handcrafted Features

S. Arunmozhi[1], *Vaddi Satya Sai Sarojini*[2], *T. Pavithra*[3], *Varsha Varghese*[3], *V. Deepti*[3], *and V. Rajinikanth*[3]

[1]Department of Electronics and Communication Engineering, Manakula Vinayagar Institute of Technology, Puducherry, 605 107, India

[2]Department of Information Technology, St. Joseph's College of Engineering, Chennai600 119, Tamil Nadu, India

[3]Department of Electronics and Instrumentation Engineering, St. Joseph's College of Engineering, Chennai600 119, Tamil Nadu, India

CONTENTS

DOI: 10.1201/9781003198796-11

11.1 INTRODUCTION

Recently, the incidence of diseases in humans is rapidly rising due to a variety of reasons. Based on the spread, the diseases are classified into (i) communicable and (ii) noncommunicable diseases. The noncommunicable disease will affect only a person and this disease can be treated using an appropriate medication. But, communicable diseases cause a serious problem to a larger human group and also increase the morbidity and the mortality rate when the uncontrolled disease spreads to a larger group [1–7].

From the literature, it is known that the spread of infectious disease among people is very common and if the spread affects a large human community globally, then it is called a pandemic. Even though a considerable number of infectious diseases are widely found globally; the infection due to novel coronavirus (COVID-19) rapidly infected a wider population globally and because of its infection as well as the spread rate, COVID-19 was declared a pandemic in early 2020 [8,9].

The earlier research on COVID-19 confirmed that it leads to severe pneumonia in humans and the unnoticed and untreated disease will cause casualty. Hence, a number of preventive and precautionary ways are suggested and applied globally to control the spread of the disease. Further, the following research works are also implemented: detection of protein structure of the virus, disease modelling to predict the progress of the disease, sample-assisted detection procedure, image-based infection level detection, and controlling methodology for the infection using prescribed drug [10–13].

The commonly adopted COVID-19 detection methodologies are as follows: (i) sample collection from the suspicious patient, (ii) RT-PCR test for the initial level confirmation, (iii) image-assisted infection level assessment, and (iv) treatment planning and execution to cure the patient. In the abovementioned method, the image-assisted COVID-19 diagnosis plays a major role in most of the hospitals; in which the radiological procedures, such as the Computed-Tomography (CT) and the Chest Radiographs (X-ray) are recorded and evaluated. The radiological images captured using a chosen technique are evaluated by an experienced radiologist and the doctor using a personal check as well as the computer-assisted imaging technique and based on the report and the suggestion, the essential treatment procedure is planned and implemented to cure the patient. Literature confirms that the assessment of COVID-19 infection using lung CT is widely preferred [14–16].

The aim of this research is to implement an automated segmentation system to examine the test image. This work implements the modern segmentation procedure developed using the CNN to extract the stained fragment in lung CT. The proposed technique implements the following procedures: (i) image resizing, (ii) saliency detection, (iii) CNN-based segmentation, (iv) extraction of classical features, (v) dominant feature selection with Bat-algorithm (BA), and (vi) classification and validation.

During the experimental investigation, benchmark lung CT images with COVID-19 infection are used for the assessment and the proposed investigational work is executed using the resized images with dimension 572 × 572 × 1 pixels. The CNN-based segmentation procedure called the VGG-UNet is employed to extract the infected fragment. The texture features, such as GLCM and Hu moments, are then extracted and the dominant features are then selected using the Bat-algorithm (BA). The selected features are used to train, test, and validate the two-class classifier and the performance is then validated based on the classification accuracy.

The proposed research work is prearranged as: Section 11.2 describes the context, Section 11.3 presents the methodology, and Sections 11.4 and 11.5 depict the results and discussions and the conclusions, respectively.

11.2 EARLIER RESEARCH

Due to its significance, recently, research with image-assisted COVID-19 detection is proposed by researchers using the chest radiographs and the lung CT scan images. The lung CT scan slices will offer a better diagnosis compared to the chest

TABLE 11.1
Summary of the Earlier COVID-19-Related Work Implemented with Lung CT

Research work	Implemented Assessment Technique
Ahuja et al. [17]	Propose a DL system to examine the disease using the lung CT slices. In this work, the performance of the well-known DL systems are compared and the proposed work confirms that the DL architecture helps attain a classification accuracy >98%.
Dey et al. [18]	Propose a ML technique to examine the COVID-19 disease using lung CT slices. This work realized a hybrid processing scheme to extract the infected fragment from the test image and this method helped accomplish a classification accuracy of >87% with the KNN classifier.
Ardakani et al. [19]	This work developed a dedicated COVID-19 system named COVIDiag; which helps detect the infected sections from the lung CT scan images with better detection accuracy.
Ardakani et al. [20]	This work presented a detailed assessment of ten most successful deep-learning schemes to detect the COVID-19 lesion from the lung radiology images.
Joshi et al. [21]	Detailed discussion of the computer assisted automated detection of the pneumonia infection from the patients is presented.
Khan et al. [22]	This work implemented the deep-learning supported detection of the COVID-19 using the optimally selected features. A detailed assessment with a two class and multi class classifier is presented and the proposed work is authenticated with other methods.
Rajinikanth et al. [23]	This work presented a semi-automated assessment to extract and evaluate the COVID-19 lesion in 2D slices. This work also presented a methodology to assess the severity of the COVID-19 lesion infection area and lung area.
Rajinikanth et al. [24]	Automated extraction and evaluation of the COVID-19 lesion from the lung CT image is presented. This work employed a heuristic algorithm-assisted segmentation.

radiographs and the earlier research works proposed and implemented with the lung CT scan images are summarized in Table 11.1. Most of the earlier works implemented the machine-learning (ML) and the deep-learning (DL) systems to examine the COVID-19 infection with better classification accuracy.

In literature, a number of COVID-19 detection and forecasting approaches are already proposed and implemented to efficiently detect/predict the infection [12,25].

This work implements CNN-based joint segmentation and classification technique to examine the 2D lung CT images. The motivation is to efficiently classify the test images into normal/COVID-19 class using binary classifiers. In this work, only the handcrafted features along considered and the dominant features are selected using the BA. The classification task implemented with the SVM-RBF helped in achieving a better result than other considered classifiers.

11.3 METHODOLOGY

The methodology employed to examine the COVID-19 infection with the proposed scheme is described in Figure 11.1. The considered image is 3D and in order to reduce the computation burden, 3D to 2D conversion is implemented and the converted image is then considered for the COVID-19 assessment. In this work, the VGG-UNet is considered to segment the COVID-19 lesion from the considered test image. The VGG-UNet accepts only the images with dimension 572 × 572 × 1 pixels and hence an image alteration is applied to adjust the dimension of the test image based on the need. After the resizing, an image saliency detection technique is employed to identify the Region of Interest (ROI) from the trial image. The saliency detection technique will identify the COVID-19 section to be extracted from the trial image. When the perfectly trained VGG-UNet is implemented on the test image, it will mine the COVID-19 disease from the test image. The essential image features from the extracted infection is then mined using the GLCM and the Hu moments and then the dominant features are

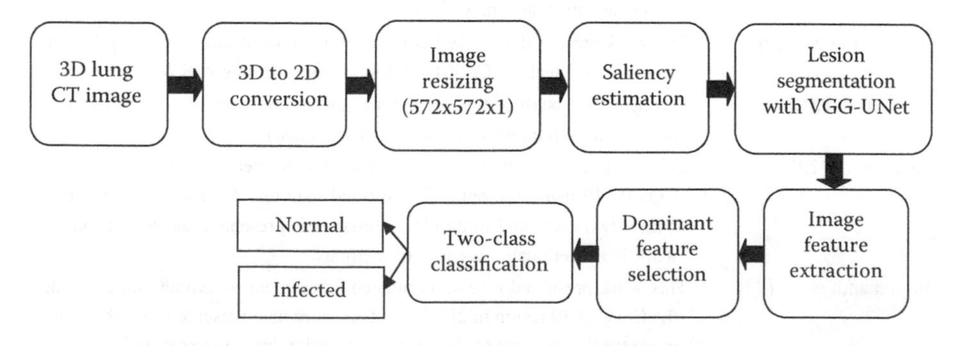

FIGURE 11.1 Structure of the Proposed COVID-19 Segmentation and Classification Scheme.

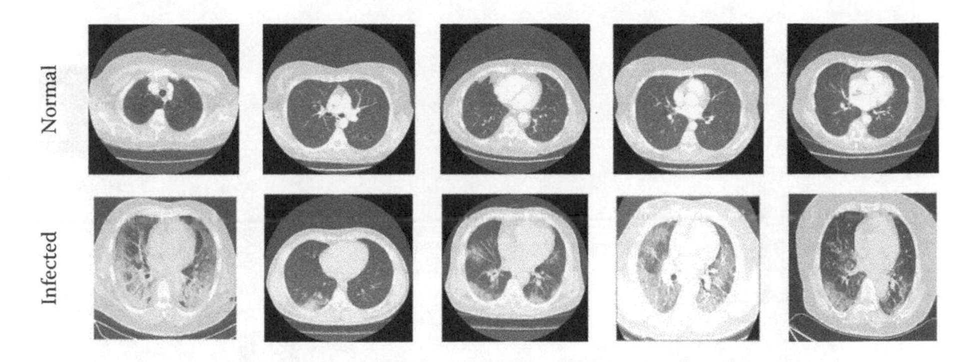

FIGURE 11.2 Sample Test Images Considered in the Proposed Research Work.

then selected using the BA-based feature selection technique. The chosen features are adopted to train, test, and validate the two-class classifiers.

11.3.1 Image Database

To promote the research and to find the solution for problems in COVID-19 detection, copyright-free lung CT images are made available for the research community and in the proposed work, the lung CT images (normal/infection) are collected from CT dataset [26]. This dataset consists 3D CT images along with its GT and to decrease the computation burden, the 3D images are converted into 2D slices and all the considered images are then resized into 572 × 572 × 1 pixels. Figure 11.2 depicts the sample test images considered for the experimental investigation and in this work; the considered segmentation methodology is implemented to extract the COVID-19 lesion from the considered lung CT images. The total images considered in every case are presented in Table 11.2.

11.3.2 Segmentation with VGG-UNet

In medical image assessment task, segmentation plays a critical role and in most of the cases, a preferred segmentation system is implemented to extort the ROI for further evaluation. In the literature, traditional semi-automated and automated

TABLE 11.2
Lung CT Slices Considered in the Proposed Research Work

Category	Pixel Dimension	Total CT Images	Number of Images for Training	Number of Images for Validation
Normal	572 × 572 × 1	1,000	700	300
Infected	572 × 572 × 1	1,000	700	300

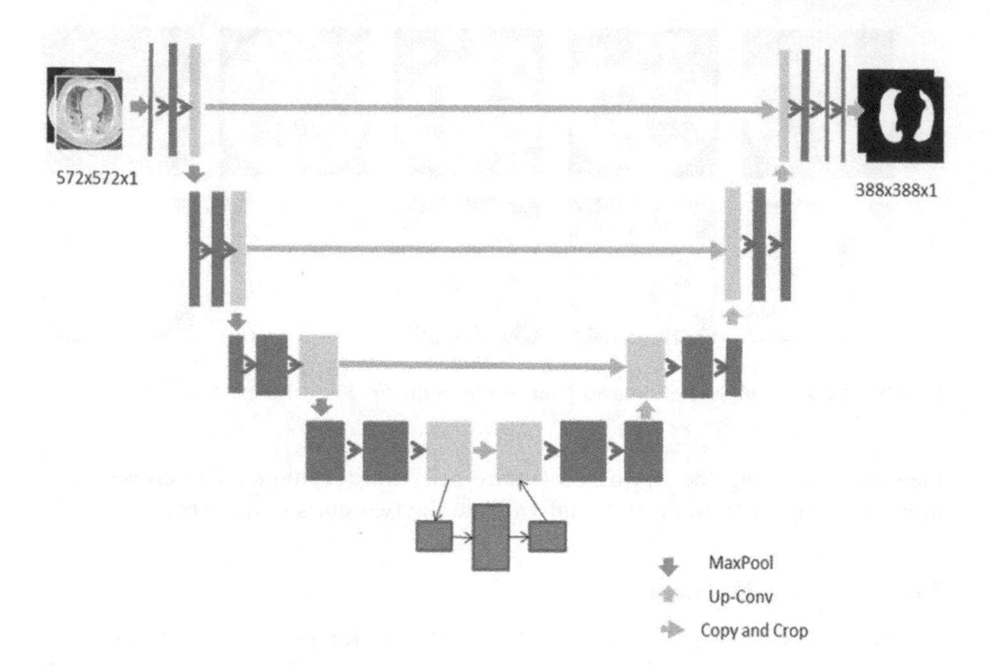

FIGURE 11.3 VGG-UNet Architecture Employed in the Proposed Work.

practices are extensively employed to extract and evaluate the ROI from the chosen medical grade images [27–32]. The traditional segmentation needs operator's assistance and most of the traditional methodology also requires the image preprocessing tasks. To overcome the problem, recently, the CNN-based segmentation procedures are widely adopted by the researchers [33–39].

Figure 11.3 depicts the conventional VGG-UNet architecture, widely employed to extort ROI [40–44]. The various stages of the proposed CNN segmentation is clearly presented in Figure 11.3 and this architecture helps extort the ROI (COVID-19 disease) with better segmentation accuracy. The earlier works implemented with this scheme confirms the superiority of VGG-UNet segmentation and in the proposed work; this scheme is employed to extort the COVID-19 infection from the chosen test image. The final layer of the proposed scheme offers a binary version of the image with a dimension of 388 × 388 × 1 and this image is then considered for the extraction of the image features, which further helps categorize test images into normal/infection group.

11.3.3 Feature Extraction

The earlier works related to automated disease classification using a chosen medical image modality confirm that the feature extraction and feature-assisted classification is the prime task in the disease detection task. In this work, the essential image features, such as Gray Level Co-occurrence Matrix (GLCM) and the Hu are extracted from the binary version of the ROI. The implemented technique helped to extract 34 numbers of features (25 GLCM features + 9 Hu moments) from the binary image. The existing features in this image are quite large and if all these features are used; we may face a overfitting problem. To avoid this, it is necessary to select the dominant feature set using a suitable statistical and modern test. The statistical test is time consuming and hence the BA is applied to select the essential feature set using the carefully selected GLCM and Hu moments [45–52].

11.3.4 Feature Selection with Bat Algorithm

The number of raw features accessible for each image case is large and if these features are used without any additional treatment, the problem of over-fitting will happen. To avoid this, a feature-reduction or a dominant feature-selection technique is implemented and this technique helps reduce the available raw features to a lower level. Feature reduction using a traditional statistical technique is time-consuming and hence, heuristic algorithm-based methods are extensively adopted by the researchers to identify the dominant features during the automated disease detection process. In this work, BA-assisted feature choosing technique is employed to reduce image features. The working of BA is extensively discussed in the literature and the BA algorithm considered here computes the Cartesian distance among the features and select the features; whose distance is more and the BA considered in this work can be accessed from [53–55].

The BA-based feature reduction implemented in this work is shown in Figure 11.4 and this process helped to lessen the 1 × 1 × 34 features into 1 × 1 × 7 features used to test the classifiers.

11.3.5 Classifier Implementation

The classifiers play a chief role in disease recognition with machine learning and the deep learning systems. In the proposed work, the commonly used customary categorization routines, such as Decision-Tree (DT), Random-Forest (RF), K-Nearest

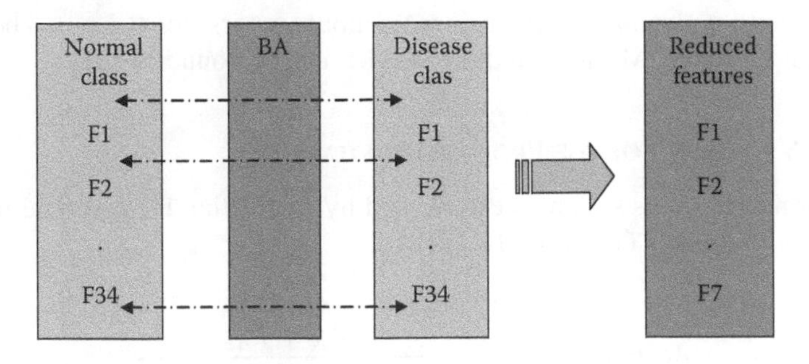

FIGURE 11.4 BA-assisted Feature Reduction Technique.

Neighbor (KNN), SVM-Linear, and SVM-RBF are considered to divide the existing picture dataset into normal/disease classes.

11.3.5.1 Decision-Tree

DT is one if the extensively used classifiers related for the linear/nonlinear features with a succession of assessment design which progress in the shape of a tree-like flow graph and the related information is found in [45,47].

11.3.5.2 Random-Forest

RF is an enhanced process and very vigorous to noise and competent on considerable datasets. It specified as a set of tree interpreters. Every tree is relying on an arbitrary vector, which are sampled separately and allotted in such a way that the tree is distributed in the forest. The classical RF technique is widely used in various image classification tasks [45,47].

11.3.5.3 K-Nearest Neighbor

KNN approximates the space from a series of new information to all training data points, and discovers the direct coldness as the best neighbor. The k significance is empirically computed by means of the training sample's organization error. The other information on KNN can be found in [47,48].

11.3.5.4 SVM-RBF

SVM is one of the famous classifiers in image examination field and in SVM; the data are alienated into assessment exterior, which imply the hyperplane and its supply also to exploits the margins among classes by treating the data in a nonlinear fashion.

The decision function of SVM is

$$C(a) = Sgn\left[\sum_{i=1}^{Nv} b_i \in i.\, K(s_i, a) + y\right] \tag{11.1}$$

where $\in i$ are the Lagrange coefficient acquired through the optimization development.

The separating plane is created using Nv input-vectors, for $\in i \neq 0$. The related information on the SVM-linear and SVM-RBF can be found in [51].

11.3.6 Validation of the Proposed System

The performance of this system is established by calculating the essential measures presented in Equations (11.2) to (11.7) [51,52]:

$$Accuracy = ACC = \frac{T_{+ve} + T_{-ve}}{T_{+ve} + T_{-ve} + F_{+ve} + F_{-ve}} \tag{11.2}$$

$$Precision = PRE = \frac{T_{+ve}}{T_{+ve} + F_{+ve}} \tag{11.3}$$

$$Sensitivity = SEN = \frac{T_{+ve}}{T_{+ve} + F_{-ve}} \tag{11.4}$$

$$Specificity = SPE = \frac{T_{-ve}}{T_{-ve} + F_{+ve}} \tag{11.5}$$

$$F1Score = F1S = \frac{2T_{+ve}}{2T_{+ve} + F_{-ve} + F_{+ve}} \tag{11.6}$$

$$Negative Predictive Value = NPV = \frac{T_{-ve}}{T_{-ve} + F_{-ve}} \tag{11.7}$$

where F_{+ve}, F_{-ve}, T_{+ve}, and T_{-ve} signify false-positive, false-negative, true-positive, and true-negative, respectively.

11.4 RESULTS AND DISCUSSIONS

This section presents and discusses the investigational outcome.

The stages depicted in Figure 11.1 are employed in the proposed work using the resided 2D slice of the lung CT and the following results are attained. Initially, this scheme is implemented on the normal class lung CT images and no segmentation result is attained with the VGG-UNet for the normal class lung CT case. When the similar methodology is implemented with the lung CT images associated with the COVID-19 infection, the proposed CNN segmentation procedure effectively extracts the infected section with better accuracy.

Figure 11.5 depicts the typical result of the normal and the infected class lung CT image; in which Figure 11.5(a) to (c) presents the chosen test image, saliency map, and the extracted ROI, respectively. This image also confirms that, for the normal image class, the VGG-UNet fails to extract the ROI since, in this image category, no ROI is applicable. For the infected image case, the ROI will be the COVID-19 lesion, which is then effectively extracted with the proposed segmentation approach.

Comparable practice is repeated on all the images of this study (1,000 normal and 1,000 infected class) and from each image, the essential image features are extorted using the GLCM and the Hu. The essential image features are then selected with the BA (1 × 1 × 7 features) and the selected features are considered to test classifiers. In this work, 70% of images (700 numbers) of each class are used to train the classifier and 30% of images (300 numbers) are to validate the classifiers.

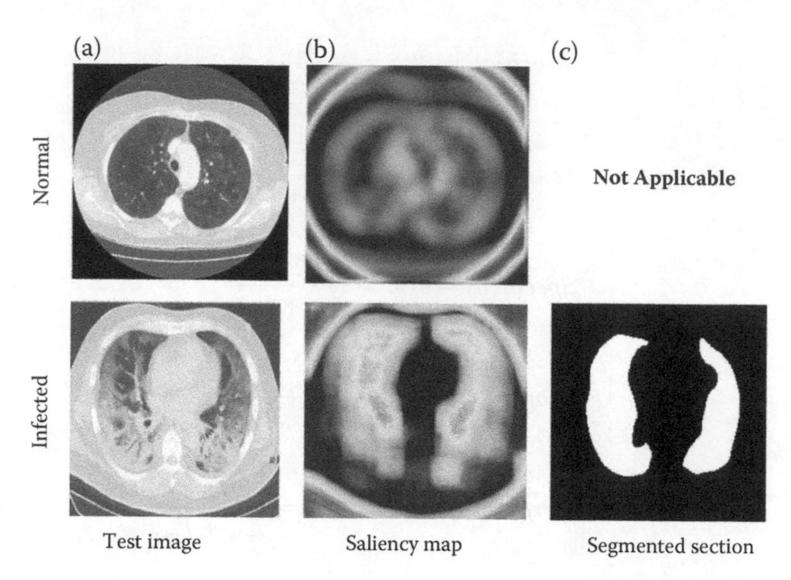

FIGURE 11.5 Results Attained with the VGG-UNet with Various Image Classes (a) Test image, (b) Saliency map, (c) Segmented section.

The performance of this scheme is computed by calculating the essential measures and the attained performance values for proposed study are depicted in Table 11.3. A five-fold cross validation is implemented during classification with all the seven features and the best value attained among the five-fold cross validation is then considered to validate the eminence of the proposed scheme.

Before the classification, an experimental investigation is employed to identify the essential number of features for the classification task and in this work, the feature size varies from 2 to 7 and the optimal number of features, which offers the best classification accuracy, is then identified. Figure 11.6 depicts the identification of the optimal features for the C = SVM-RBF and this figure confirms that, when

TABLE 11.3
Attained Performance Measures

Classifier	Optimal Features	TP	FN	TN	FP	Performance Measure (%)					
						ACC	PRE	SEN	SPE	F1S	NPV
DT	6	287	13	274	26	93.50	91.69	95.67	91.33	93.64	95.47
RF	4	275	25	283	17	93.00	94.18	91.67	94.33	92.90	91.88
KNN	5	288	12	281	19	94.83	93.81	96.00	93.67	94.89	95.90
SVM-Linear	6	278	22	281	19	93.17	93.60	92.67	93.67	93.13	92.74
SVM-RBF	5	286	14	292	8	96.33	97.28	95.33	97.33	95.42	96.29

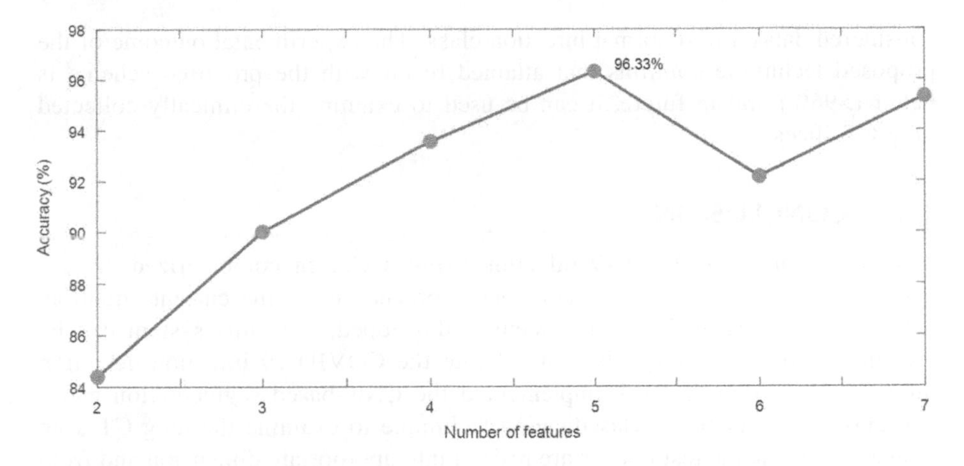

FIGURE 11.6 Comparison of the Classifier Performance with Varied Feature Values (SVM-RBF).

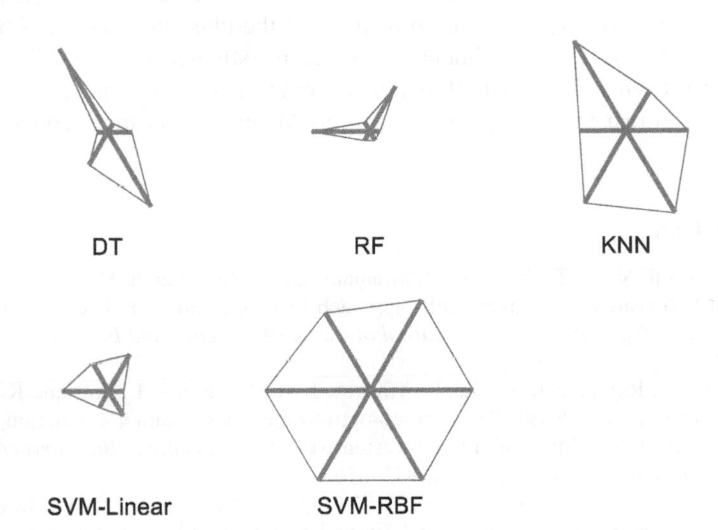

FIGURE 11.7 Glyph Plot to Confirm the Overall Performance of the Considered Classifier.

the chosen classifier dimension is 5, then the attained accuracy (96.33%) is better. Comparable practice is repeated for other classifiers and the attained outcomes are depicted in Table 11.3 (Figure 11.7).

Table 11.3 depicts the attained performance measure values with each classifier and to identify the overall performance, a Glyph plot is then constructed and this plot corroborate that the overall result by SVM-RBF is superior.

In this work, CNN segmentation is primarily employed to extort the infected section and later a two-class classifier is then executed to segregate the considered dataset into normal/infection class. The experimental outcome of the proposed technique confirms that attained result with the proposed scheme is better (>96%) and in future, it can be used to examine the clinically collected lung CT slices.

11.5 CONCLUSION

Assessment of the COVID-19 infection using a chosen computerized disease detection procedure is one of the essential procedures in the current situation. When an appropriate detection system is developed, then this system can be recommended to the hospitals to accelerate the COVID-19 infection detection process. The proposed work implemented the CNN-based segmentation and a two-class classifier-based classification technique to examine the lung CT scan images. Initially, the test images are resized into appropriate dimension and from the infected lung CT images, the COVID-19 disease is extorted using the VGG-UNet structure. The essential features are then extracted from the segmented image and then $1 \times 1 \times 7$ dimension feature vector is formed with the help of the BA. This feature vector is then used to prepare the classifier system adopted in the proposed work. The experimental work is investigated using MATLAB and attained result with SVM-RBF classifier presented better classification accuracy (>96%) in contrast to DT, RF, KNN, and SVM-linear classifiers considered in this study.

REFERENCES

[1]. Lakshmi, V. S., Tebby, S. G., Shriranjani, D., & Rajinikanth, V. (2016). Chaotic cuckoo search and Kapur/Tsallis approach in segmentation of T. cruzi from blood smear images. *International Journal of Computer Science and Information Security (IJCSIS)*, *14*, 51–56.

[2]. Dey, N., Rajinikanth, V., Shi, F., Tavares, J. M. R., Moraru, L., Karthik, K. A.,... & Emmanuel, C. (2019). Social-group-optimization based tumor evaluation tool for clinical brain MRI of Flair/diffusion-weighted modality. *Biocybernetics and Biomedical Engineering*, *39*(3), 843–856.

[3]. Wang, Y., Shi, F., Cao, L., Dey, N., Wu, Q., Ashour, A. S.,... & Wu, L. (2019). Morphological segmentation analysis and texture-based support vector machines classification on mice liver fibrosis microscopic images. *Current Bioinformatics*, *14*(4), 282–294.

[4]. Rajinikanth, V., Satapathy, S. C., Dey, N., Fernandes, S. L., & Manic, K. S. (2019). Skin melanoma assessment using Kapur's entropy and level set—A study with bat algorithm. In *Smart intelligent computing and applications* (pp. 193–202). Springer, Singapore.

[5]. Fernandes, S. L., Tanik, U. J., Rajinikanth, V., & Karthik, K. A. (2020). A reliable framework for accurate brain image examination and treatment planning based on early diagnosis support for clinicians. *Neural Computing and Applications*, *32*(20), 15897–15908.

[6]. Fernandes, S. L., Rajinikanth, V., & Kadry, S. (2019). A hybrid framework to evaluate breast abnormality using infrared thermal images. *IEEE Consumer Electronics Magazine*, *8*(5), 31–36.
[7]. Satapathy, S. C., & Rajinikanth, V. (2018). Jaya algorithm guided procedure to segment tumor from brain MRI. *Journal of Optimization, 2018.*
[8]. Zhao, D., Yao, F., Wang, L., Zheng, L., Gao, Y., Ye, J.,... & Gao, R. (2020). A comparative study on the clinical features of COVID19 pneumonia to other pneumonias. *Clinical Infectious Diseases*, *71*(15), 756–761.
[9]. Iba, T., Levy, J. H., Connors, J. M., Warkentin, T. E., Thachil, J., & Levi, M. (2020). The unique characteristics of COVID19 coagulopathy. *Critical Care*, *24*(1), 1–8.
[10]. Bhapkar, H. R., Mahalle, P. N., Dey, N., & Santosh, K. C. (2020). Revisited COVID19 mortality and recovery rates: Are we missing recovery time period?. *Journal of Medical Systems*, *44*(12), 1–5.
[11]. Shinde, G. R., Kalamkar, A. B., Mahalle, P. N., Dey, N., Chaki, J., & Hassanien, A. E. (2020). Forecasting models for coronavirus disease (COVID19): A survey of the state-of-the-art. *SN Computer Science*, *1*(4), 1–15.
[12]. Fong, S. J., Li, G., Dey, N., Crespo, R. G., & Herrera-Viedma, E. (2020). Composite Monte Carlo decision making under high uncertainty of novel coronavirus epidemic using hybridized deep learning and fuzzy rule induction. *Applied Soft Computing*, 106282.
[13]. Fong, S. J., Li, G., Dey, N., Crespo, R. G., & Herrera-Viedma, E. (2020). Finding an accurate early forecasting model from small dataset: A case of 2019-ncov novel coronavirus outbreak. arXiv preprint arXiv:2003.10776.
[14]. Kadry, S., Rajinikanth, V., Rho, S., Raja, N. S. M., Rao, V. S., & Thanaraj, K. P. (2020). Development of a machine-learning system to classify lung CT scan images into normal/COVID19 class. arXiv preprint arXiv:2004.13122.
[15]. Ambikapathy, B., & Krishnamurthy, K. (2020). Mathematical modelling to assess the impact of lockdown on COVID19 transmission in India: Model development and validation. *JMIR Public Health and Surveillance*, *6*(2), e19368.
[16]. Rauf, H. T., Lali, M. I. U., Khan, M. A., Kadry, S., Alolaiyan, H., Razaq, A., & Irfan, R. (2021). Time series forecasting of COVID19 transmission in Asia Pacific countries using deep neural networks. *Personal and Ubiquitous Computing*, 1–18.
[17]. Ahuja, S., Panigrahi, B. K., Dey, N., Rajinikanth, V., & Gandhi, T. K. (2020). Deep transfer learning-based automated detection of COVID19 from lung CT scan slices. *Applied Intelligence*, 1–15. doi: 10.1007/s10489-020-01826-w.
[18]. Dey, N., Rajinikanth, V., Fong, S. J., Kaiser, M. S., & Mahmud, M. (2020). Social-group-optimization assisted Kapur's entropy and morphological segmentation for automated detection of COVID19 infection from computed tomography images. *Cognitive Computation*, *12*, 1011–1023. doi: 10.1007/s12559-020-09751-3.
[19]. Ardakani, A. A., Acharya, U. R., Habibollahi, S., & Mohammadi, A. (2021). COVIDiag: A clinical CAD system to diagnose COVID19 pneumonia based on CT findings. *European Radiology*, *31*(1), 121–130.
[20]. Ardakani, A. A., Kanafi, A. R., Acharya, U. R., Khadem, N., & Mohammadi, A. (2020). Application of deep learning technique to manage COVID19 in routine clinical practice using CT images: Results of 10 convolutional neural networks. *Computers in Biology and Medicine*, 103795.
[21]. Joshi, A., Dey, N., & Santosh, K. C. (2020). Intelligent systems and methods to combat COVID19. *SpringerBriefs in Computational Intelligence*, 978–981.
[22]. Khan, M. A., Kadry, S., Zhang, Y. D., Akram, T., Sharif, M., Rehman, A., & Saba, T. (2020). Prediction of COVID19-pneumonia based on selected deep features and

one class Kernel extreme learning machine. *Computers & Electrical Engineering*, 106960.

[23]. Rajinikanth, V., Dey, N., Raj, A. N. J., Hassanien, A. E., Santosh, K. C., & Raja, N. (2020). Harmony-search and otsu based system for coronavirus disease (COVID19) detection using lung CT scan images. arXiv preprint arXiv:2004.03431.

[24]. Rajinikanth, V., Kadry, S., Thanaraj, K. P., Kamalanand, K., & Seo, S. (2020). Firefly-algorithm supported scheme to detect COVID19 lesion in lung CT scan images using Shannon entropy and Markov-random-field. arXiv preprint arXiv:2004.09239.

[25]. Fong, S. J., Dey, N., & Chaki, J. (2020). *Artificial intelligence for coronavirus outbreak*. SpringerLink, United States.

[26]. MosMed. (2020). *Artificial intelligence in radiology*. https://mosmed.ai/en/ (Accessed on 10.12.2020).

[27]. Dey, N., Zhang, Y. D., Rajinikanth, V., Pugalenthi, R., & Raja, N. S. M. (2021). Customized VGG19 architecture for pneumonia detection in chest X-rays. *Pattern Recognition Letters*, *143*, 67–74. doi: 10.1016/j.patrec.2020.12.010.

[28]. Kadry, S., Rajinikanth, V., Raja, N. S. M., Hemanth, D. J., Hannon, N. M., & Raj, A. N. J. (2021). Evaluation of brain tumor using brain MRI with modified-moth-flame algorithm and Kapur's thresholding: A study. *Evolutionary Intelligence*, 1–11.

[29]. Rajinikanth, V., Priya, E., Lin, H., & Lin, F. (2021). *Hybrid image processing methods for medical image examination*. CRC Press, United States.

[30]. Shree, T. V., Revanth, K., Raja, N. S. M., & Rajinikanth, V. (2018). A hybrid image processing approach to examine abnormality in retinal optic disc. *Procedia Computer Science*, *125*, 157–164.

[31]. Dey, N., Rajinikanth, V., & Hassanien, A. E. (2020). An examination system to classify the breast thermal images into early/acute DCIS class. In *Proceedings of International Conference on Data Science and Applications* (pp. 209–220). Springer, Singapore.

[32]. Rajinikanth, V., Raja, N. S. M., & Satapathy, S. C. (2016). Robust color image multi-thresholding using between-class variance and cuckoo search algorithm. In *Information systems design and intelligent applications* (pp. 379–386). Springer, New Delhi.

[33]. Badrinarayanan, V., Kendall, A., & Cipolla, R. (2017). Segnet: A deep convolutional encoder-decoder architecture for image segmentation. *IEEE Transactions on Pattern Analysis and Machine Intelligence*, *39*(12), 2481–2495.

[34]. Kendall, A., Badrinarayanan, V., & Cipolla, R. (2015). Bayesian segnet: Model uncertainty in deep convolutional encoder-decoder architectures for scene understanding. arXiv preprint arXiv:1511.02680.

[35]. Badrinarayanan, V., Handa, A., & Cipolla, R. (2015). Segnet: A deep convolutional encoder-decoder architecture for robust semantic pixel-wise labelling. arXiv preprint arXiv:1505.07293.

[36]. Tang, P., Liang, Q., Yan, X., Xiang, S., Sun, W., Zhang, D., & Coppola, G. (2019). Efficient skin lesion segmentation using separable-Unet with stochastic weight averaging. *Computer Methods and Programs in Biomedicine*, *178*, 289–301.

[37]. Weng, Y., Zhou, T., Li, Y., & Qiu, X. (2019). Nas-unet: Neural architecture search for medical image segmentation. *IEEE Access*, *7*, 44247–44257.

[38]. Li, X., Chen, H., Qi, X., Dou, Q., Fu, C. W., & Heng, P. A. (2018). H-DenseUNet: Hybrid densely connected UNet for liver and tumor segmentation from CT volumes. *IEEE Transactions on Medical Imaging*, *37*(12), 2663–2674.

[39]. Wang, C., MacGillivray, T., Macnaught, G., Yang, G., & Newby, D. (2018). A

two-stage 3D Unet framework for multi-class segmentation on full resolution image. arXiv preprint arXiv:1804.04341.
[40]. Shi, J., Dang, J., Cui, M., Zuo, R., Shimizu, K., Tsunoda, A., & Suzuki, Y. (2021). Improvement of damage segmentation based on pixel-level data balance using VGG-Unet. *Applied Sciences*, *11*(2), 518.
[41]. Yang, Y., Xu, Y., Shen, W., & Qiu, F. (2018, October). Multi-classifier detection of lung nodules based on convolutional neural network. In *2018 International Conference on Image and Video Processing, and Artificial Intelligence* (Vol. 10836, p. 108361F). International Society for Optics and Photonics, USA.
[42]. Balakrishna, C., Dadashzadeh, S., & Soltaninejad, S. (2018). Automatic detection of lumen and media in the IVUS images using U-Net with VGG16 encoder. arXiv preprint arXiv:1806.07554.
[43]. Liu, L., & Zhou, Y. (2018, August). A closer look at U-net for road detection. In *Tenth International Conference on Digital Image Processing (ICDIP 2018)* (Vol. 10806, p. 108061I). International Society for Optics and Photonics, USA.
[44]. Liu, J., Wang, X., & Wang, T. (2019). Classification of tree species and stock volume estimation in ground forest images using Deep Learning. *Computers and Electronics in Agriculture*, *166*, 105012.
[45]. Jahmunah, V., Oh, S. L., Rajinikanth, V., Ciaccio, E. J., Cheong, K. H., Arunkumar, N., & Acharya, U. R. (2019). Automated detection of schizophrenia using nonlinear signal processing methods. *Artificial Intelligence in Medicine*, *100*, 101698.
[46]. Rajinikanth, V., Raja, N. S. M., & Kamalanand, K. (2017). Firefly algorithm assisted segmentation of tumor from brain MRI using Tsallis function and Markov random field. *Journal of Control Engineering and Applied Informatics*, *19*(3), 97–106.
[47]. Acharya, U. R., Fernandes, S. L., WeiKoh, J. E., Ciaccio, E. J., Fabell, M. K. M., Tanik, U. J.,... & Yeong, C. H. (2019). Automated detection of Alzheimer's disease using brain MRI images–a study with various feature extraction techniques. *Journal of Medical Systems*, *43*(9), 302.
[48]. Khan, M. A., Kadry, S., Alhaisoni, M., Nam, Y., Zhang, Y., Rajinikanth, V., & Sarfraz, M. S. (2020). Computer-aided gastrointestinal diseases analysis from wireless capsule endoscopy: A framework of best features selection. *IEEE Access*, *8*, 132850–132859.
[49]. Bakiya, A., Kamalanand, K., Rajinikanth, V., Nayak, R. S., & Kadry, S. (2020). Deep neural network assisted diagnosis of time-frequency transformed electromyograms. *Multimedia Tools and Applications*, *79*(15), 11051–11067.
[50]. Rajinikanth, V., Dey, N., Kavallieratou, E., & Lin, H. (2020). Firefly algorithm-based Kapur's thresholding and Hough transform to extract leukocyte section from hematological images. In *Applications of firefly algorithm and its variants* (pp. 221–235). Springer, Singapore.
[51]. Rajinikanth, V., Joseph Raj, A. N., Thanaraj, K. P., & Naik, G. R. (2020). A customized VGG19 network with concatenation of deep and handcrafted features for brain tumor detection. *Applied Sciences*, *10*(10), 3429.
[52]. Bhandary, A., Prabhu, G. A., Rajinikanth, V., Thanaraj, K. P., Satapathy, S. C., Robbins, D. E.,... & Raja, N. S. M. (2020). Deep-learning framework to detect lung abnormality–A study with chest X-Ray and lung CT scan images. *Pattern Recognition Letters*, *129*, 271–278.
[53]. Dey, N., & Rajinikanth, V. (2020). *Applications of bat algorithm and its variants*. Springer, Singapore.
[54]. Rajinikanth, V., Dey, N., & Kavitha, S. (2020). Multi-thresholding with Kapur's

entropy—A study using bat algorithm with different search operators. In *Applications of bat algorithm and its variants* (pp. 61–78). Springer, Singapore.
[55]. Dey, N., Rajinikanth, V., Lin, H., & Shi, F. (2020). A study on the bat algorithm technique to evaluate the skin melanoma images. In *Applications of bat algorithm and its variants* (pp. 45–60). Springer, Singapore.

Index